my PILATES guru

Your ultimate pilates instructor

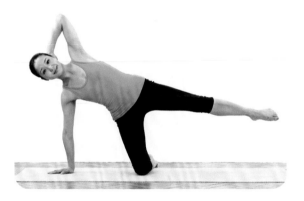

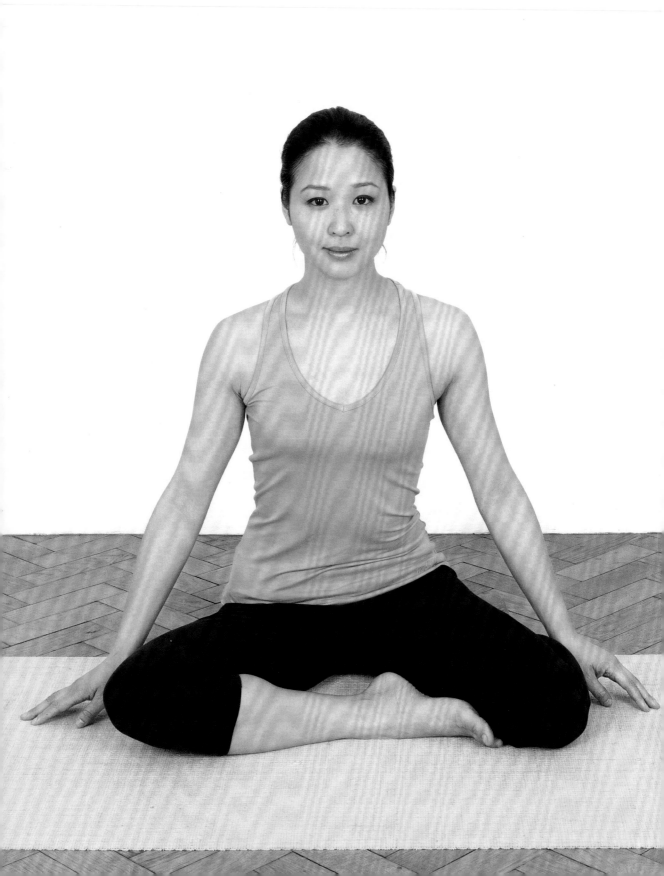

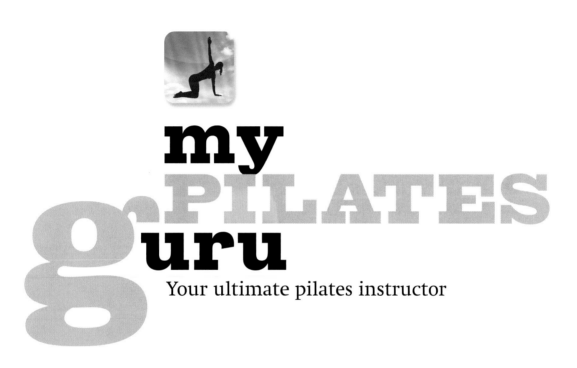

my PILATES guru

Your ultimate pilates instructor

ANYA HAYES

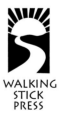

WALKING
STICK
PRESS

hamlyn

Published in the U.S. by Walking Stick Press,
an imprint of F+W Media, Inc. 10151 Carver Road,
Suite #200, Blue Ash, OH 45242
(800) 289-0963

First published in Great Britain in 2012 by Hamlyn,
a division of Octopus Publishing Group Ltd
Endeavour House
189 Shaftesbury Avenue
London
WC2H 8JY

www.octopusbooks.co.uk

ISBN 978-1-59963-622-1

A CIP catalogue record for this book is available from the
British Library.

Printed and bound in China.

10 9 8 7 6 5 4 3 2 1

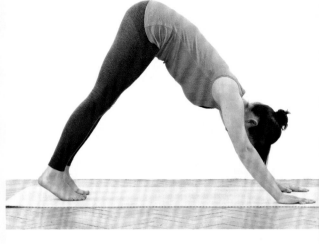

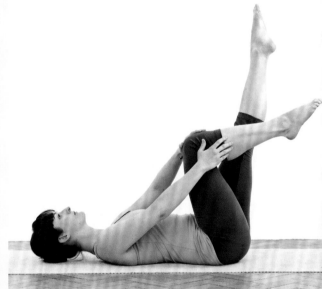

Disclaimer
Any information given in this book is not intended to be taken
as a replacement for medical advice. Any person with a
condition requiring medical attention should consult a
qualified medical practitioner or therapist before beginning
any of the postures in this book. Whilst the advice and
information in this book is believed to be accurate and the
advice, instruction, or formulae have been devised to avoid
strain, neither the author nor the publisher will be responsible
for any injury, losses, damages, actions, proceedings, claims,
demands, expenses and costs (including legal costs or
expenses) incurred or any way arising out of following the
exercises in this book.

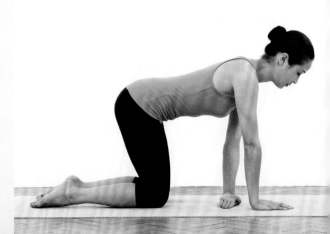

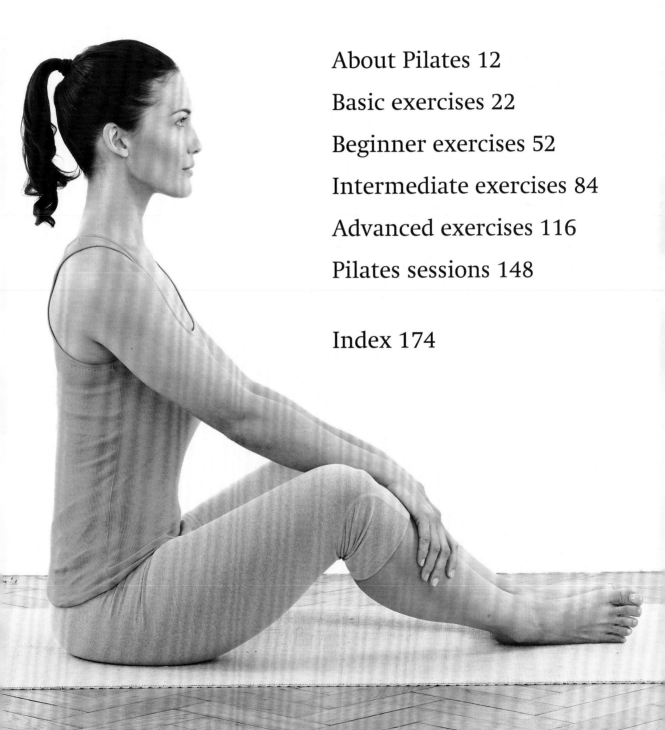

Contents

Introduction 6

About Pilates 12

Basic exercises 22

Beginner exercises 52

Intermediate exercises 84

Advanced exercises 116

Pilates sessions 148

Index 174

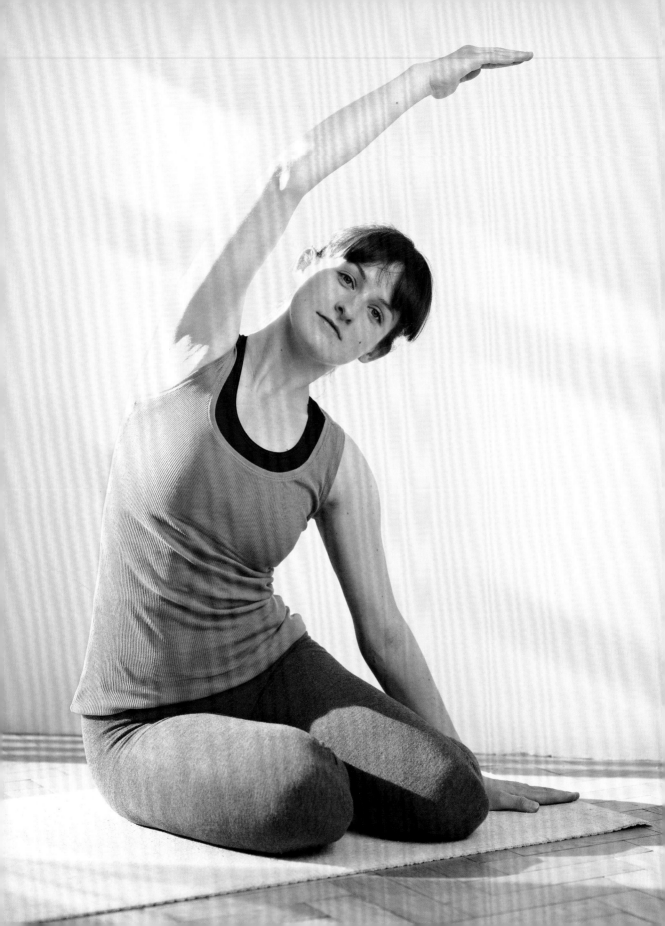

Introduction

The fact that you have picked up this book shows that you are interested in the health of your body and forms of movement, and want to find inspiration for your fitness regime. You won't be disappointed! By committing to taking up Pilates you have already started on a journey to better health and wellbeing. With regular practice, you'll become better aligned and better coordinated; you'll walk taller and your movement will be more graceful; your balance will improve and your breathing will be deeper and more effective. On top of all of this, you will shape your waist and your limbs will become a longer and leaner as your muscles tone up. People will ask you if you've been on holiday, you will seem so fresh faced and relaxed.

The Pilates way

Pilates is a fantastic body-conditioning programme that is dynamic, challenging and playful. Every workout will be as effective as the amount of focus and work you put in, so use this book to become your own personal trainer and encourage your competitive side – try to build on your progression steadily and advance your own development. This book gives you the tools not only to learn how to do Pilates, but also to learn how to hone the detail of your skills to get the most out of your workout. You can incorporate the Pilates principles into your daily life, making it a truly cross-training discipline that delivers amazing results, sculpting your body and awakening your mind.

My Pilates Guru opens up the world of Pilates for you so that whether you are a first-time exerciser or a seasoned gym-goer, you will be able to find the level of challenge for you. It first takes you through the basics, giving you a strong foundation for your Pilates journey by describing the fundamental principles and

movements to get you started. It then builds up layers of challenge in the beginner, intermediate and advanced exercise sections. Regular Pilates practitioners can dive straight in with the intermediate or advanced sections, but you are encouraged to mix it up and revisit the basics regularly so that you can perfect your technique as well as the overall effectiveness of your practice.

Each section offers the chance to vary certain exercises according to your ability: you can make a beginner's exercise more difficult, and an advanced exercise less challenging. There is also a guru guide for each exercise, outlining what to take particular care over while you are performing the exercise.

Towards the end of the book you are shown how to create your own workout programmes, drawing from all sections and which you can tailor to your own needs and desires. It's time to get started!

How to use My Pilates Guru

My Pilates Guru is a meticulously structured guide to the world of Pilates. Taking you from the basics through to advanced exercises and ending with specifically designed sessions, each element ensures you are perfectly equipped for best practice.

Introducing My Pilates Guru

About Pilates (see pages 12–21) explains the main principles behind Pilates, focusing on movements of the spine, alignment, breathing and posture.

Basic exercises (see pages 22–51) contains a selection of Pilates matwork exercises that form the basic platform of your Pilates practice, ranging from the relaxation position and neutral pelvis and spine to centring (see below) and spinal movements.

Three further chapters of exercises – beginner (see pages 52–83), intermediate (see pages 84–115) and advanced (see pages 116–47) – explore the Pilates repertoire from the simplest of exercises to the most strenuous. Whatever the level, you are led by the hand to maximize your potential (see opposite, top).

Pilates sessions (see pages 148–73) designed for you to explore in different ways (see opposite, bottom) round off the book.

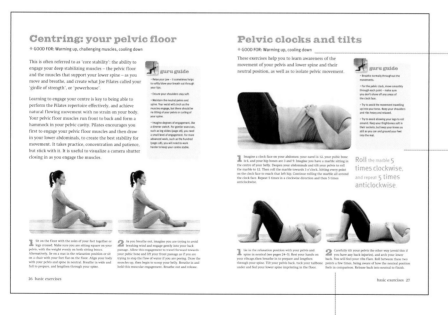

• This information explains the core purpose of each exercise. Use it, too, to create your own workouts (see pages 150–3).

• GURU GUIDE
Advice for enhancing your skills is given for each exercise in handy bite-sized snippets.

Starting off

The first two chapters set the scene. Revisit them frequently to remind yourself how to get the most from the exercises described in subsequent chapters.

• STEP TEXT AND PICTURES
Broken down into steps, you are led through Pilates technique to achieve the optimum position.

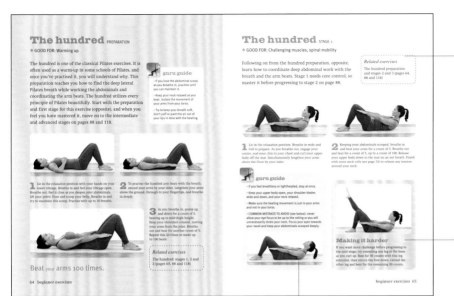

RELATED EXERCISES
Many Pilates exercises are divided into stages. To help you find your way around the book, page numbers for further stages are given for relevant exercises.

MAKING IT HARDER
Once you've mastered an exercise, you may wish to push yourself that little bit further before moving on to the next level.

Pilates exercises

Each aspect of Pilates technique is carefully explained for every exercise. They are ordered sequentially within appropriately levelled chapters, as for a Pilates workout.

COMMON MISTAKES TO AVOID
To get the most from Pilates you must be correctly aligned. Pictures like this show you what NOT to do.

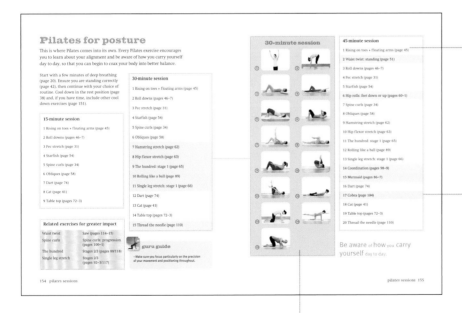

LENGTH OF TIME OF SESSION
To help you fit Pilates into your life, different lengths of session are given. You can also choose to start with the shortest session and build it up to a longer length of time.

GREY PANEL IN SESSIONS BOXES
These show you where more exercises have been added to build them up from what has gone before. If you want to use exercises that will give you even greater impact, use the 'Related exercises' box, opposite.

Pilates sessions

Carefully crafted sessions that focus on specific parts of the body or time of day and to various lengths of time are given on pages 154–73.

PHOTO PANEL
Pictures for each exercise in one routine (here, for the 30-minute session) act as a memory aid.

Your free App

My Pilates Guru is designed to be a complete package. It comes with a free iPhone application that is downloadable from iTunes. With this application you will be able to:

- View exercises.
- Create your own sessions.
- View pre-loaded or saved sessions.
- Monitor your progress and record your development.

Downloading the App

To download the App, simply go to the App Store and type in 'My Pilates Guru'. The App you want has the 'My Guru' logo (right).

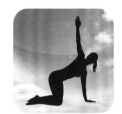

My Pilates Guru

Note: you can download the application for either iPhone or iPad and it is compatible with any version.

The App is simple to use and follow. After the title screen you will be given a number of options:

1. Introduction

This explains how best to use the application and how to navigate your way around its menus and features.

2. All Exercises

Here you can view all the exercises in the book together with their variations. You can search the exercises in different ways:

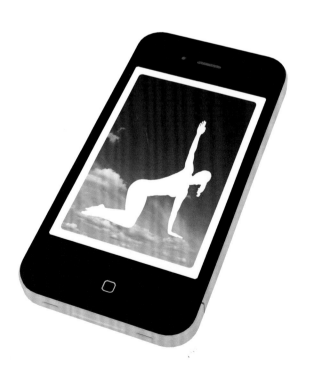

- Those that are good for a particular thing, such as flexibility or joints.
- Skill level: beginner, intermediate or advanced.
- Those you've marked as favourite.
- By keyword.

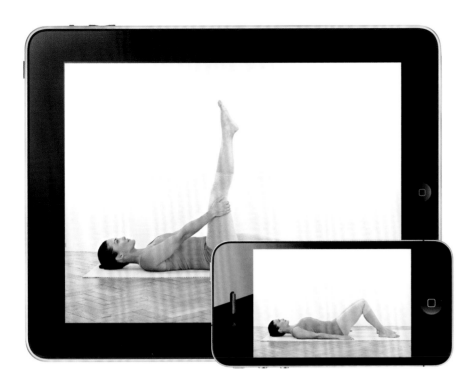

Each individual exercise screen shows you what skill level it is suitable for. It also has options to add the exercise to a session, mark it as a favourite or even share the fact you're doing it on social media.

Tapping on the image will allow you to see photographs of the steps of that exercise. These images are a memory aid only. Always refer to the book should you want specific step-by-step instruction.

3. Sessions

This is where you can build your own Pilates sessions, save them, or follow the samples at the back of this book (see pages 149–173). All the session examples from the book are here, so you've no need to build them yourself. The 'My sessions' tab will allow you to bring up the saved sessions, adapt them and rename them should you require.

For more advice about how to best structure your Pilates sessions, refer to pages 150–153. Don't forget to hit the 'I've done this session' button at the end of every session so that your activity is recorded.

4. My results

This part of the App records the sessions you've completed so that you can monitor your progress over time by level and what the exercises are good for. You can also see which exercises and sessions you use the most and monitor your weight and body mass index. This is a superb way to see the benefits of your My Guru experience as your skills develop.

5. About My Gurus

This section gives you updated information about the latest books and packages available in the series.

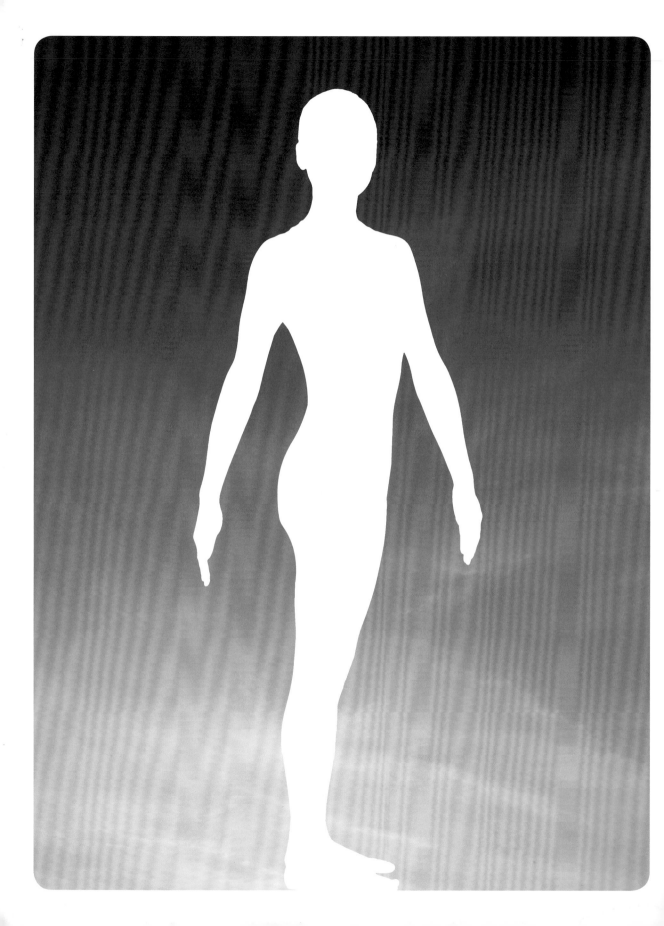

About Pilates

Welcome to your guru guide to Pilates. In this section
you will learn about the fundamental principles of Pilates
and what makes it such a wonderful body-conditioning
programme. In this chapter you will look at the core
benefits of Pilates, together with muscle balance,
alignment and breathing.

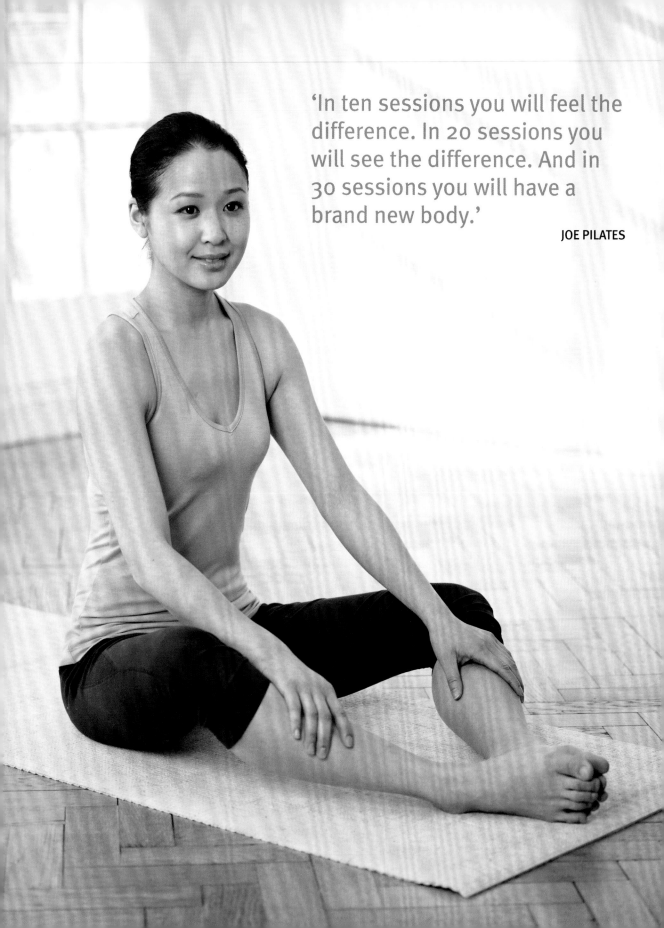

'In ten sessions you will feel the difference. In 20 sessions you will see the difference. And in 30 sessions you will have a brand new body.'

JOE PILATES

The origins of Pilates

The Pilates method was developed by Joseph Hubertus Pilates, known as Joe to all who followed him. Born in Germany in 1880, he was a sickly child, suffering from rickets, rheumatic fever and asthma. As a result, when he grew older he became obsessed with physical fitness and improving his body image. He studied anatomy and trained as a body builder, gymnast and boxer, drawing inspiration from martial arts and yoga. He was ahead of his time, believing that the 'modern' lifestyle full of 'automobiles and fast living', combined with bad posture and poor breathing, were the main causes of ill health.

The Pilates system was born

Joe Pilates was living in England, working as a circus performer and boxer, when he was placed in forced internment because of his nationality at the outbreak of the First World War. While in internment, he began to develop an exercise system to help rehabilitate bedridden injured soldiers. After the War, Pilates returned to Germany. He had developed a reputation as a physical trainer and, in 1925, he was asked to use his exercise system to train the German Army. Reluctant to allow what he felt was an indomitable body-conditioning programme to be used to benefit the increasingly right-wing regime, he packed his bags and took a boat to New York City, where he met his future wife Clara. He went on to establish his studio in New York with her, and developed an exercise method he named Contrology, which evolved into what we now know as Pilates.

At his New York studio, Pilates' clients were originally boxers, but he happened to be working in the same building as a number of dance studios, and it wasn't long before the boxers were driven out by leading ballet dancers. Dancers began to depend on Pilates training for the strength and grace it developed, as well as for its rehabilitative effects of easing muscle pains and preventing injuries.

Joe Pilates died in 1967 as a result of a fire in his studio, and he was remarkably robust physically right up until the end of his life. He is also said to have had a flamboyant personality, and was an intimidating teacher. He loved cigars, and liked to show off his impressive physique, always wearing nothing but tight exercise briefs in his studio. Joe Pilates' teachings were carried on by those who trained directly with him in New York, known as the Pilates Elders, who spread his work beyond New York City and throughout the world. Some committed themselves to passing along Joe's work exactly as he taught it, often called 'classical style' Pilates. Other students went on to develop the exercises with their own teaching styles. The method continues to be developed today.

The principles of Pilates

There are six principles that Pilates originally applied to his body-conditioning programme. Applied to your practice they will create balance, grace and ease of movement, while you exercise and in your daily life.

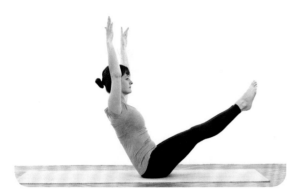

Centring: The energy of Pilates comes from your centre, what Joe Pilates called your 'powerhouse' or 'girdle of strength'. This is the muscular area between your ribcage and pelvis, supporting the spine, referred to throughout as the abdominals. This deep muscle strength supports your body in movement.

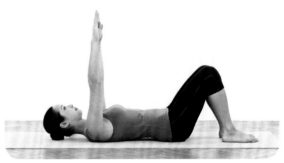

Precision: Precise execution of each movement and correct alignment is key to the effectiveness of Pilates, and requires patience and practice. At first, precise alignment and movement requires deep concentration, but with regular practice it will become natural.

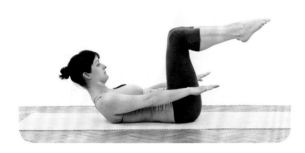

Breath: Joe Pilates said, 'Squeeze out the lungs as you would wring a wet towel dry. Soon the entire body is charged with fresh oxygen from toes to fingertips.' Synchronizing the use of the breath to the movement is a fundamental aspect of Pilates.

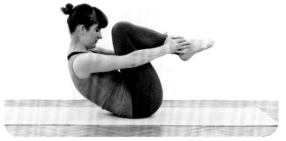

Flowing movements: When practising Pilates, repeat each sequence with continuous, flowing movement, synchronized with the breath. Pilates movements are even-paced and fluid, lengthening out from a strong centre and mobilizing your joints fully.

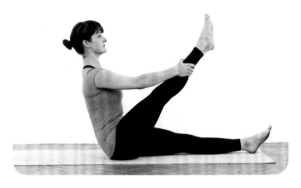

Concentration: Pilates requires concentration and deep focus – there should be no mindless repetition in which your body runs on autopilot. Practising Pilates you will develop body awareness and control, through concentration on the detail and precision of the movement. This mental connection to your body allows you to release unwanted tension and encourages a deep sense of relaxation.

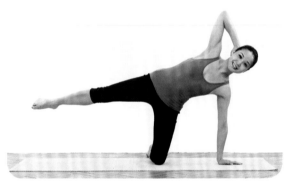

Control: Pilates strengthens by using controlled movements, using gravity and your own body weight as resistance – the slower the movement, the harder you have to work. Every exercise requires muscular and mental control to develop an awareness of each part of your body being involved in the exercise, even if it is not moving. This enables you to work the targeted muscles while maintaining your breathing and alignment, and ensure no unnecessary tension.

The benefits of Pilates

Pilates is an unbeatable body-conditioning programme that develops strength, tone and body awareness. It combines strengthening with relaxation, and the physical and mental benefits are manifold. Pilates encourages natural elegance and grace every day, not simply while exercising. The exercises lighten the load on your spine and joints by correcting muscular imbalances and posture, and alleviating unnecessary muscle tension.

You rediscover your body's natural movement patterns, restoring balance lost by bad posture, lack of use or misuse of muscles. The result is a beautiful freedom of movement of your limbs and strength of spine, which feels wonderful and has the fantastic by-product of making you look taller, leaner and more poised as well.

Performing the exercises slowly makes them more challenging for the muscles. With continued and regular practice of Pilates, you will achieve:

► A firmer, flatter stomach together with a defined waist
► Improved posture
► Toned arms, shoulders, back, buttocks and thighs
► Increased flexibility
► More efficient breathing and better blood circulation
► Improved core strength and coordination
► More energy
► Greater bone density
► Relief from muscle tension and any back pain you may suffer from.

Movements of the spine

Pilates ensures the muscles in your body are balanced – no part of your body is ignored or focused on at the detriment of others. The focus of a Pilates workout is equally on both sides of the body, front to back, top to bottom, and based on the ideal symmetry of alignment and natural movement. This helps to correct imbalances caused by bad posture or muscle stress, releasing over-dominant muscles and strengthening underused muscles. You are encouraged to mobilize all of your joints fully and take your spine safely through every aspect of potential movement, as illustrated here.

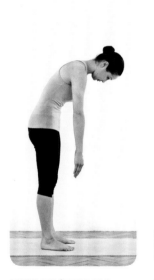

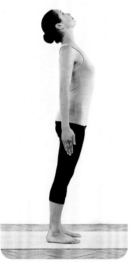

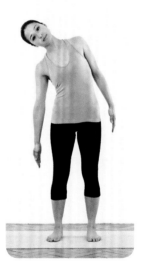

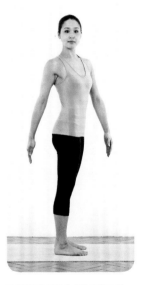

FLEXION (BENDING FORWARD)

EXTENSION (BENDING BACKWARDS)

LATERAL FLEXION (SIDE BENDING)

ROTATION (TWISTING)

Balancing your workout

A balanced workout will include all of these movements as equally as possible, to ensure the spine has been fully mobilized and the muscles on the front and back of the body have been equally strengthened and released (for more information, see pages 150–3). Some of the exercises go further, by combining two elements of spinal movement, for example rotation with flexion in oblique curl ups (see page 58).

Alignment

Proper alignment balances your skeleton as it was designed to be, so that your muscles are held at their ideal length and strength, and there is no tension and strain anywhere. Good alignment helps to reduce the impact that gravity has on your body, spine and joints, whether you are moving or still. The Pilates workout is therefore an opportunity to learn to correct your misalignments and imbalances and achieve the optimal placing of your muscles. In time you will feel the benefits of improved posture, more efficient joint mobility and improved circulation. Joe Pilates felt that muscular balance and perfect skeletal alignment was key to overall vitality.

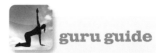

guru guide

• As you exercise, always be aware of your alignment as it will impact on the effectiveness of the movement performed and, particularly with the more dynamic exercises, will lessen the chance of strain or injury.

• While exercising, use a mirror where possible to check your alignment and develop your awareness of where your body is in space.

Symmetry in Pilates

Make use of the mat as a guide for your symmetry and placing. Try not to be sitting or standing on it crookedly. Instead, ensure you are working in the centre and measure the distance of the sides and ends of the mat from your body, and then try to keep these distances equal as you proceed through the exercises in your workout.

In addition to checking your alignment when standing, you also need to be aware of neutral pelvis and spine (see page 25) as well as your alignment when lying on the mat (see page 24).

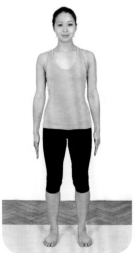

◀ Your head should be directly in the centre of your shoulders.

◀ Your shoulders should be level and arms released by your sides, palms facing in towards your thighs.

◀ Your hips should be level and your waist even on both sides.

◀ Your legs should be straight but not locked, with your weight evenly balanced on both feet.

FROM THE FRONT

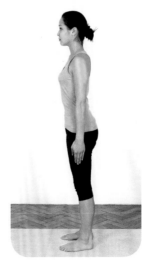

◀ Your neck should maintain its natural curves.

◀ Your ear should be in line with your shoulder.

◀ Your abdominals should be lifted inwards and upwards so that they support your spine.

◀ Feel that your head is lengthening upwards at the end of your spine.

FROM THE SIDE

Breathing

Joe Pilates was opposed to 'lazy breathing'. Coordinated, conscious and deep breathing is a fundamental aspect of Pilates practice, and often the aspect that most people struggle with at first.

Breathing is essential for life, but something we are often not conscious of, and many of us breathe shallowly and inefficiently. Pilates encourages a full lateral breath into the back of your body, so you can engage your abdominals fully while breathing deeply. The most important thing is never to hold your breath as you move as this will create tension. Keep breathing, and over time the Pilates breath will become natural as you exercise and in your daily life.

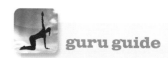

guru guide

• The benefits of deep Pilates breathing are:
– The ability to fully engage your abdominals as you exercise
– Increased lung capacity, giving you better heart and lung health
– Reduced blood pressure
– Better blood circulation, oxygenation of your muscles and organs, and glowing skin
– Greater ability to deal with stress; the act of deep breathing is relaxing.

Control your breathing

When first focusing on your breath, be aware of the way your lungs move within your ribcage during inhalation and exhalation. They are located within your ribs and open out into your back when inhaling. When practising your breathing, try to allow the exhalation to last longer than your inhalation. Count to 5 for your in breath and to 7 for your out breath to expel all the air from your lungs and encourage a natural, deep and full in breath.

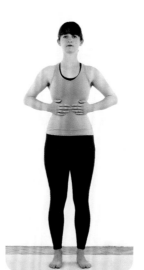

◀ As you breathe in, feel the back and sides of your ribs widening with your breath as your lungs expand.

◀ If you can only feel your chest or belly rising, you are breathing too shallowly.

◀ Try to channel your breath deeply into the back of your lungs, until you can feel your back expanding.

◀ Breathe in through your nose, making sure your shoulders stay soft and away from your ears.

INHALING

◀ As you breathe out, you will feel your ribcage soften and narrow beneath your hands.

◀ Exhale all the air out through your mouth, slowly and consciously. Sigh the breath out through your lips, relaxing your face.

◀ As you breathe in and out, concentrate on it feeling natural and not at all forced.

EXHALING

Posture

Posture is the way we hold ourselves, not only while standing but also when sitting and throughout everyday activities and movement. As noted when looking at alignment (see page 19), when your skeleton is perfectly aligned, your muscles are all at their ideal length and strength, and there is no tension and strain anywhere.

Good posture helps to reduce the impact that gravity has on your body, on your spine and your joints, every day. It also has a great impact on your wellbeing: how you carry yourself affects your physical and mental health. With ideal posture, all your vital organs are held in the right place, you have enough room to breathe, no constriction, everything functions more effectively, you move freely without aches and pains. Sounds good, doesn't it? So, what goes wrong? Think about your everyday life. Many factors influence your posture – here are a few of them.

Your job: do you sit at a desk all day? Drive a lot? Holding your body in a certain way for over 8 hours a day will, over time, affect your muscle balance.

Illnesses or injuries affect the way you carry yourself.

Hobbies/sport you play can create muscle imbalances, any types of repetitive movements over time mean that you hold your body in a certain way.

Emotional issues: if you are depressed you are likely to show this in your posture.

Fashion: do you wear high heels every day? Or if you are a very tall woman, you may, without realizing, allow your posture to slump so as not to bring attention to your height.

The beauty of Pilates is that you soon take its posture principles into your everyday life. With practice, your muscles will be more evenly balanced and you will sit and walk taller, you will breathe more deeply and your circulation will improve.

Posture check

• Do a quick posture check every day, as you are standing waiting for the bus, or sitting at your desk ... wherever you are.

• Are your shoulders relaxed into your back rather than slumped forward? Try to draw them softly into your back and lengthen your spine.

• Is your weight even on both feet?

• Are your hips level?

• If you are sitting, are you slumped into your lower back?

• Where is your tailbone? Lengthen it down and release the crown of your head up to the ceiling. Lift your pelvis away from your hips to activate the deep supporting muscles around your lower spine and your pelvic floor.

• Try to encourage yourself into ideal alignment every day, and look to rectify any postural habits that you have (see page 42).

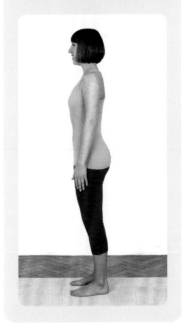

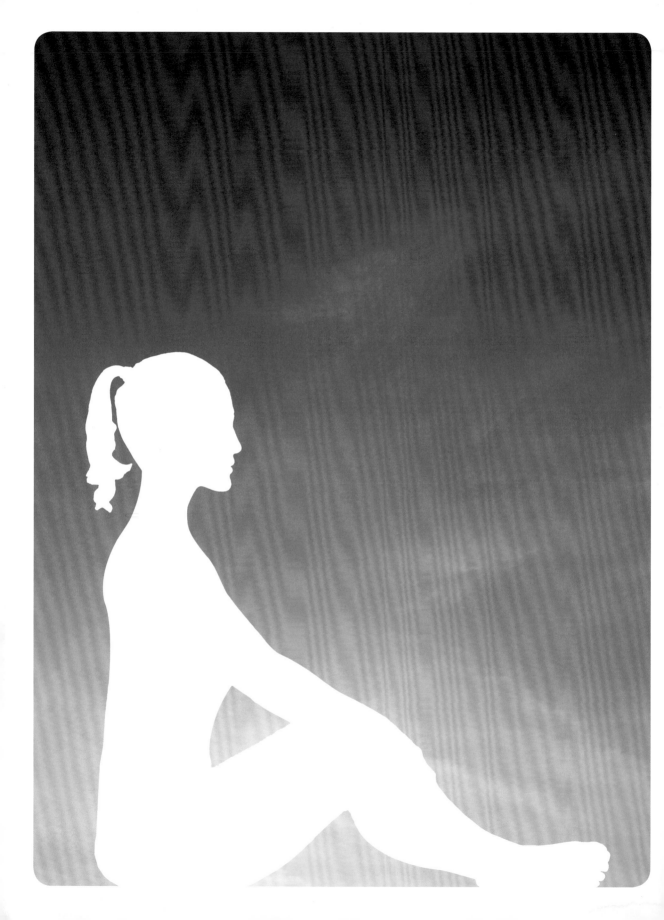

Basic exercises

In this section there is a selection of Pilates matwork exercises that form the basic platform of your Pilates practice. These exercises are suitable for anyone who is new to Pilates, as well as being an important reminder of the general principles and patterns of movement for anyone who is familiar with the programme. Mastering the basics enables you to get the most out of the more challenging exercises later on. Practise and perfect them, and continue to revisit these exercises even as you progress through the programme.

Relaxation position

◆ GOOD FOR: Warming up, cooling down

This is a wonderful position for finding your neutral spine and to encourage release of muscle tension. It is a common starting position for many exercises.

Lie on a mat, with a firm pillow underneath your head if your posture requires it. You should feel relaxed around your neck and shoulders, and your eye gaze directed to the ceiling, your head neither tipped forward nor back. Place your feet flat on the floor, in parallel and in line with your hips, with your knees bent. Have your arms by your sides with palms flat to the floor, lengthening out through your fingertips.

Be aware of the points of contact on the floor: around the back of your head, shoulders, ribcage, tailbone and feet. Release through each point. Breathe in deeply and feel your ribcage widening in the mat. Breathe out to soften and relax. Continue to breathe fully. Release your body into the mat, let your weight surrender to gravity and soften your muscles.

Become aware of any areas of tension and allow them to soften into the floor. Feel your collarbones widen and hip joints soften. Feel your thighbone deepening into its socket and the back of your tailbone heavy and released. Be aware of your feet, softening your toes into the floor so they are grounded.

guru guide

• Feel the support of the floor under your body. Notice how your body feels rather than collapsing your weight into the floor.

• Imagine you are lying on wet sand and think about the imprint your body would make in the sand.

• Soften your jaw, release your tongue from the roof of your mouth and make sure the muscles of your face are released and shoulders wide and full.

• Let your spine lengthen into its natural curves – imagine a small space opening between each vertebra.

• If you are using this as a relaxation at the end of the day, place your hands on your lower belly to release fully through the back of your shoulders.

Let your weight surrender to gravity.

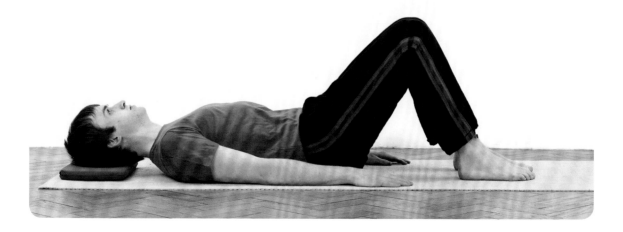

Neutral pelvis and spine

◆ GOOD FOR: Warming up, cooling down

Neutral alignment of your pelvis and spine is a position you need to find to perform all the exercises in this book. It encourages balance in your muscles and releases tension in your lower back.

Lie on a mat, in the relaxation position (see opposite). Breathe in deeply and place your hands on your ribcage to feel your ribcage widening. To find neutral position, release your arms by your sides. Visualize a triangle shape of your pubic and hip bones. Try to feel they are level and parallel with the floor.

Bring your awareness to your spine. Feel its curves releasing into the mat. Notice which body parts are heavy on the mat, and which are lighter or not touching. With your spine in neutral, you will feel the back of your head on the mat (or pillow), and lifted through the back of your neck. You will be heavy around your shoulders and anchored around your ribcage. Your lower back will be lifted slightly in its natural curve. Relax it.

Check with your hands that you can gently fit your fingers under your spine into this natural curve – this is a guide only, it will depend on your body shape. Feel light in this part of your spine, as your tailbone again is heavy and grounded. Your feet should feel evenly placed and heavy.

guru guide

• Imagine your pelvis is a bowl of water resting on the floor: the water level should be flat, not tilting and spilling on any side.

• COMMON MISTAKES TO AVOID: if you can feel your lower spine imprinting in the mat (see below), you are not in neutral pelvis or spine – your pelvis has tilted back and you have lost the natural curve. If you are arched in your back with a big space under your lower spine, your pelvis may have rocked out of neutral.

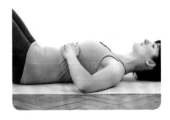

Feel light in this part of your spine.

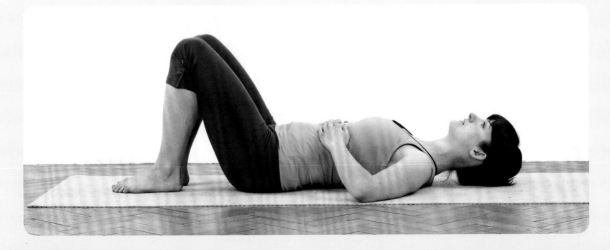

Centring: your pelvic floor

◆ GOOD FOR: Warming up, challenging muscles, cooling down

This is often referred to as 'core stability': the ability to engage your deep stabilizing muscles – the pelvic floor and the muscles that support your lower spine – as you move and breathe, and create what Joe Pilates called your 'girdle of strength', or 'powerhouse'.

Learning to engage your centre is key to being able to perform the Pilates repertoire effectively, and achieve natural flowing movement with no strain on your body. Your pelvic floor muscles run front to back and form a hammock in your pelvic cavity. Pilates encourages you first to engage your pelvic floor muscles and then draw in your lower abdominals, to create the best stability for movement. It takes practice, concentration and patience, but stick with it. It is useful to visualize a camera shutter closing in as you engage the muscles.

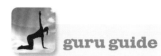

guru guide

• Relax your jaw – it sometimes helps to softly blow your breath out through your lips.

• Ensure your shoulders stay soft.

• Maintain the neutral pelvis and spine. Your waist will cinch as the muscles engage, but there should be no tilting of your pelvis or curling of your spine.

• Imagine degrees of engagement, like a dimmer switch. For gentler exercises, such as leg slides (page 28), you need a small level of engagement. For more advanced work, such as the hundred (page 118), you will need to work harder to keep your centre stable.

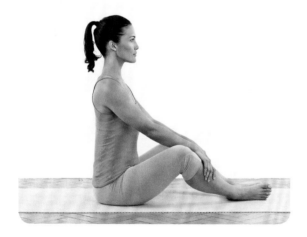

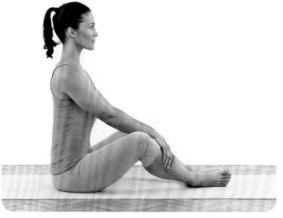

1 Sit on the floor with the soles of your feet together or legs crossed. Make sure you are sitting square on your pelvis, with the weight evenly on both sitting bones. Alternatively, lie on a mat in the relaxation position or sit on a chair with your feet flat on the floor. Align your body with your pelvis and spine in neutral. Breathe in wide and full to prepare, and lengthen through your spine.

2 As you breathe out, imagine you are trying to avoid breaking wind and engage gently into your back passage. Allow this engagement to travel forward towards your pubic bone and lift your front passage as if you are trying to stop the flow of water if you are peeing. Draw the muscles up, then begin to scoop your belly. Breathe in and hold this muscular engagement. Breathe out and release.

Pelvic clocks and tilts

◆ GOOD FOR: Warming up, cooling down

These exercises help you to learn awareness of the movement of your pelvis and lower spine and their neutral position, as well as to isolate pelvic movement.

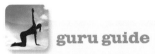

guru guide

• Breathe normally throughout the movements.

• For the pelvic clock, move smoothly through each point – make sure you don't shave off any areas of the clock face.

• Try to avoid the movement travelling up into your torso. Keep your shoulders and ribs heavy and relaxed.

• Try to avoid allowing your legs to roll around. Keep your thighbones soft in their sockets, but keep your knees as still as you can and ground your feet into the mat.

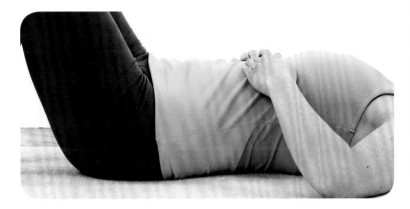

1 Imagine a clock face on your abdomen: your navel is 12, your pubic bone is 6, and your hip bones are 3 and 9. Imagine you have a marble sitting in the centre of your belly. Deepen your abdominals and tilt your pelvis to roll the marble to 12. Then roll the marble towards 3 o'clock, hitting every point on the clock face to reach that left hip. Continue rolling the marble all around the clock face. Repeat 5 times in a clockwise direction and then 5 times anticlockwise.

Roll the marble 5 times clockwise, and repeat 5 times anticlockwise.

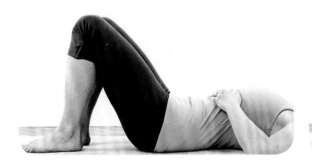

1 Lie in the relaxation position with your pelvis and spine in neutral (see pages 24–5). Rest your hands on your ribcage, then breathe in to prepare and lengthen through your spine. Tilt your pelvis back, tuck your tailbone under and feel your lower spine imprinting in the floor.

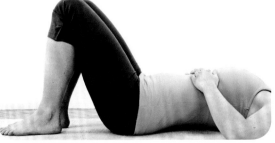

2 Carefully tilt your pelvis the other way (avoid this if you have any back injuries), and arch your lower back. You will feel your ribs flare. Roll between these two points a few times, being aware of how the neutral position feels in comparison. Release back into neutral to finish.

Leg slides

◆ GOOD FOR: Warming up, joint mobility

This exercise warms up the hip joints, and begins to challenge your core stability, requiring you to be able to control movements from a strong centre. It encourages smooth movement of the limbs while keeping your pelvis and spine in neutral.

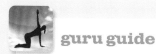

guru guide

• Maintain an engagement of your core throughout.

• Keep your waist long and even on both sides as you slide each leg away.

• Imagine you have headlights shining from your hip bones – these lights should remain shining directly up to the ceiling with the movement, they should not change direction.

Related exercise

Starfish (page 54)

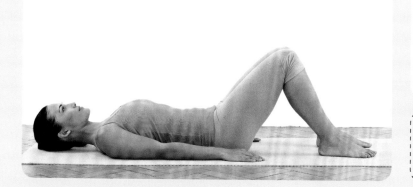

1 Lie in the relaxation position with your pelvis and spine in neutral (see pages 24–5). Release your arms down by your sides or put your hands on your hip bones if this helps guide you with the movement. Breathe in to prepare and lengthen your spine.

Repeat up to 10 times.

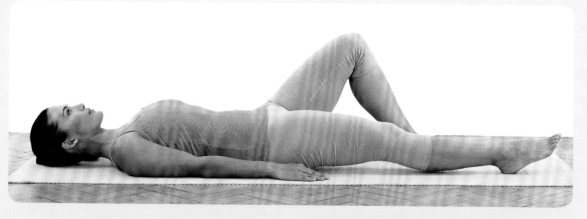

2 Breathe out and gently engage your pelvic floor and abdominals as you slide one leg away from your body, in line with your hip. Breathe in and return your leg to the bent position. Make sure your pelvis stays stable and in neutral throughout. Repeat with the other leg. Repeat up to 10 times.

Knee drops

◆ GOOD FOR: Warming up, joint mobility

A deceptively difficult exercise: this challenges your core stability and your ability to control movements from your centre. It encourages you to challenge your range of movement within your hip joint, while maintaining a neutral pelvis.

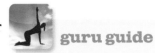

guru guide

• Feel the weight evenly on both buttocks throughout the exercise and feel anchored through both sides of your pelvis evenly.

• Focus on your thighbone moving independently of your pelvis.

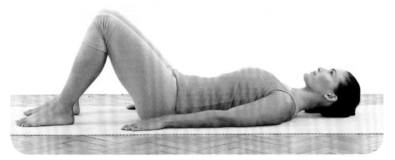

1 Lie in the relaxation position with your pelvis and spine in neutral (see pages 24–5). Release your arms down by your sides or put your hands on your hip bones if this helps guide you with the movement. Breathe in to prepare and lengthen your spine.

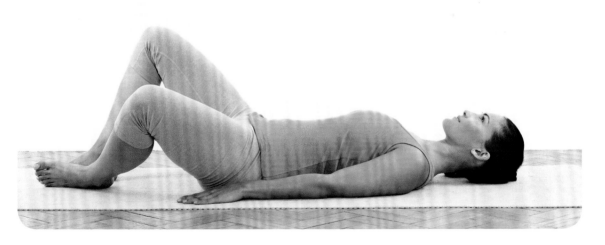

2 Breathe out, deepen your abdominals and open one knee slowly out to the side. Only go as far as you can maintain the stability of your pelvis and stay neutral – no rocking. Allow your foot to roll onto its outer edge to follow the movement of the leg, keeping your foot on the floor. Breathe in and keep your abdominals strong as you draw your knee back to the start position. Repeat with the other leg. Repeat up to 10 times on each leg.

Ribcage closure

◆ GOOD FOR: Warming up, joint mobility

A lovely exercise for releasing tension around your shoulders. It challenges your spinal stability, focusing on flowing movements.

Repeat up to **10 times.**

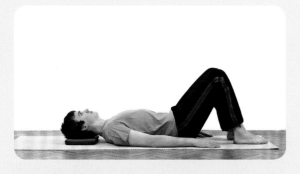

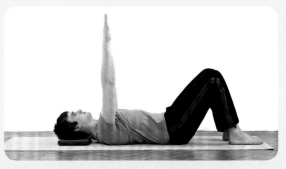

1 Align yourself in the relaxation position (see page 24). Connect to your centre, maintaining your pelvic floor and abdominal engagement throughout.

2 Breathe in to prepare and lengthen your spine. Raise your arms towards the ceiling, palms forward. Keep your elbows soft and fingertips long throughout.

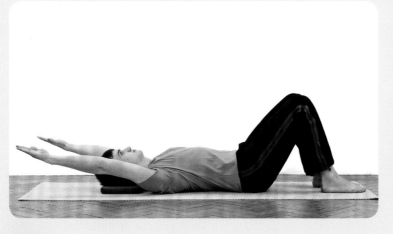

3 Breathe out, and reach both arms behind you towards the floor, keeping them in line with your ears and only go back as far as feels comfortable. Make sure your ribcage stays heavy and grounded, and do not allow your ribs to flare and your back to arch. Feel a connection from your ribs to your hips, using your abdominals. Breathe in and bring your arms back above your shoulders, allowing your chest to stay soft and open. Breathe out and lower your arms back to the mat by your sides. Repeat up to 10 times.

 guru guide

• Make sure the movement is controlled and your arms are moving simultaneously in time with each other.

• Maintain a length between your shoulders and ears – try not to allow your shoulders to rise, allow them to move naturally and freely along your ribcage.

Related exercises

Arm circles (page 32)

Spine curls with arms (page 100)

Pec stretch

◆ GOOD FOR: Warming up, stretching, cooling down

This is a great stretch to release the muscles across your chest, which can become tight due to poor posture and desk-bound jobs.

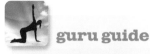
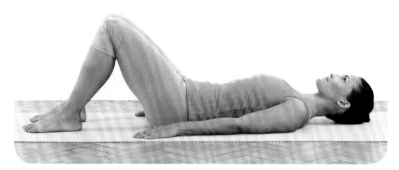

1 Align yourself in the relaxation position (see page 24). Connect to your centre, maintaining your pelvic floor and abdominal engagement throughout. Breathe in to prepare and lengthen the spine, and raise your arms up towards the ceiling, palms facing forward.

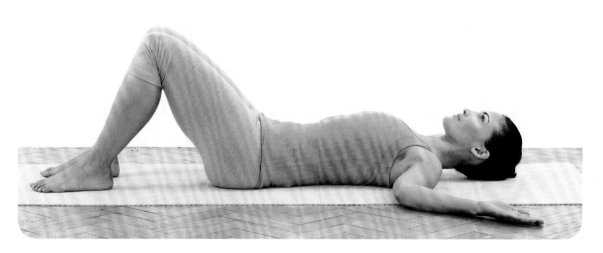

2 Breathe out and reach both arms behind you towards the floor, palms facing up. Release your arms in a wide 'V' shape, with your elbows as soft as you need to relax your arms completely to the floor without any tension and without changing the shape of your spine. Feel the front of your chest and the muscles around your armpits opening and releasing. Breathe deeply into the back of your ribcage and allow the stretch to deepen as the front of your body softens.

Arm circles

◆ GOOD FOR: Warming up, joint mobility, cooling down

This lovely exercise mobilizes your shoulders and challenges spinal stability. It also encourages flowing and controlled movement and works on your coordination.

Repeat up to 10 times in each direction.

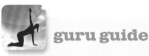

guru guide

• Stay relaxed around your neck and jaw, and maintain a space between your shoulders and ears.

• Make sure your spine does not move as your arms are circling, and ensure both your arms move at the same speed.

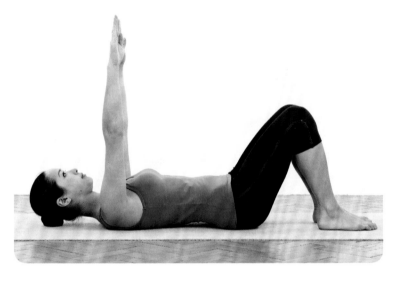

Related exercise

Double leg stretch: stage 2 (pages 120–1)

1 Align yourself in the relaxation position (see page 24). Connect to your centre, maintaining your pelvic floor and abdominal engagement throughout. Breathe in to prepare and lengthen your spine, and raise your arms up towards the ceiling, palms facing forward.

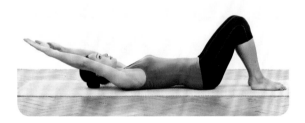

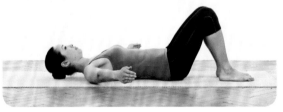

2 Breathe out and reach both arms behind you towards the floor, keeping them in line with your ears. Release your arms back only as far as feels comfortable, do not force them all the way to the floor. Feel your ribcage soft and heavy into the mat as you release your arms behind you.

3 Breathe in and circle your arms out to the side, palms facing forward. Bring your arms down by your sides once more, and turn your palms down as you reach the start position. Repeat up to 10 times, then circle your arms in the opposite direction.

Chin tucks and neck rolls

◆ GOOD FOR: Warming up, cooling down

These exercises teach you to balance the muscles around your neck and be aware of neutral alignment of your head and neck. They also release tension around your neck and shoulders, and free your neck at the end of your spine.

Repeat each exercise 8 times.

Chin tucks

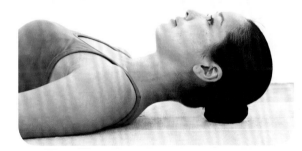

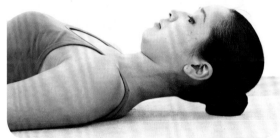

1 Align yourself in the relaxation position (see page 24). Relax your neck and jaw, free your tongue from the roof of your mouth and allow your neck to be free and long. Breathe in to prepare and lengthen your spine.

2 Breathe out and nod your chin towards your chest, keeping your head on the mat. Return to centre and breathe in to open your throat and tip your nose back slightly. Return to the centre. Repeat 8 times.

Neck rolls

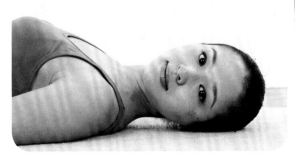

guru guide

• For greater comfort and support, place a pillow beneath the back of your head.

• Stay relaxed around your neck and jaw and maintain a space between your shoulders and ears. Feel your shoulder blades widen and melt into the floor.

• Allow your head to stay heavy on the floor; do not try to lift it and strain your neck.

1 Breathe in to prepare and as you exhale roll your head gently to one side. Bring it back to the centre and roll over to the other side, trying to encourage the same range of movement on each side. Repeat 8 times.

Spine curls

◆ GOOD FOR: Warming up, spinal mobility, cooling down

This is a lovely exercise to challenge your centre, mobilize your spine and allow you to concentrate on sequential fluid movement. It tones your buttocks wonderfully, as well as massaging your spine and releasing tension.

Related exercise

Spine curls: progression (pages 100–1)

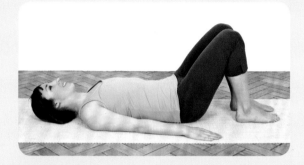

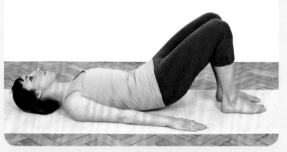

1 Lying in the relaxation position (see page 24), feel soft and open around your shoulders, ribs, tailbone and feet. Breathe in fully to prepare.

2 As you breathe out, engage your pelvic floor and tilt your pelvis back, imprinting your lower spine into the mat. Engage your buttock muscles as you begin to lift your bottom and roll your spine up off the mat, bone by bone.

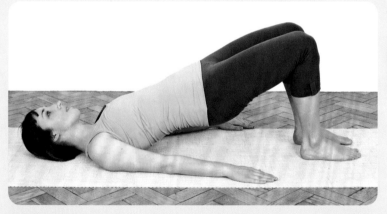

 guru guide

• COMMON MISTAKES TO AVOID (see below): try not to allow your back to arch. Deepen your abdominals, lift your buttocks, lengthen your spine and feel there is a straight line from shoulders to knees.

3 Continue to roll your spine until you feel your weight evenly across the back of your shoulder blades. Keep your knees level and hip-width apart. Keep your buttocks lifted and tailbone curled underneath you – your pubic bone should be the highest part of the torso. Feel your weight evenly on both feet and ground through all ten toes. Breathe in and maintain the length of your spine and lift of your buttocks. As you breathe out, roll your spine evenly back down to the mat, keeping your buttocks lifted for as long as possible. Breathe in at the bottom, and repeat up to 8 times.

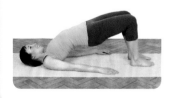

Knee folds

◆ GOOD FOR: Warming up, joint mobility, challenging muscles

Single knee folds challenge your ability to maintain a stable pelvis and spine, moving your legs independently and mobilizing your hip joint. Once you are confident with the exercise, you may vary the pace by breathing out to float your leg up, and breathing in to lower it. The double knee fold offers a greater challenge and requires a lot more core stability and abdominal strength. You will need to turn up your abdominal engagement in order to stabilize properly.

guru guide

• Make sure your pelvis and spine stay stable and in neutral.

• Keep your lower abdominals scooped; try not to allow them to bulge.

• Stay grounded and relaxed around your shoulders.

Single knee fold

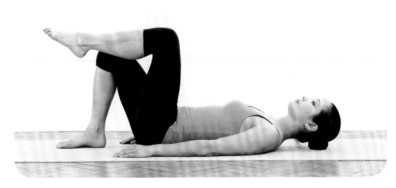

1 Align yourself in the relaxation position (see page 24), arms released by your sides. Breathe in to prepare and lengthen your spine. Breathe out, gently engage your pelvic floor and scoop your lower abdominals as you fold one knee in towards your chest. Allow your thighbone to drop into its socket and feel anchored. Make sure your shin is parallel to the floor. Breathe in to hold the position, and as you breathe out, lower your leg.

Double knee fold

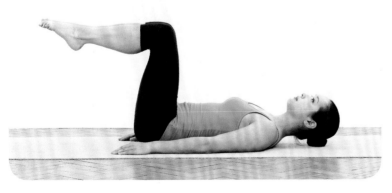

1 Float one leg in as above, and, breathe in to maintain the position. Breathe out, deepen your abdominals further and float your second knee in towards your chest, keeping your shins parallel to the floor. Breathe in to maintain the position. Breathe out, and float your first foot down, keeping your abdominals engaged. On the same out breath, return your second foot to the floor.

Prone stabilizing

◆ GOOD FOR: Warming up

This exercise allows you to find the stable and neutral position of your spine and pelvis in a front-lying position. It prepares you for the starting position in exercises such as the dart.

Related exercise
Cobra (page 104)

Align yourself centrally on your front. Create a diamond shape with your arms, opening your elbows and placing your palms down, fingertips together. Rest your forehead on the back of your hands. Position your legs hip-width apart in parallel.

Feel your tailbone lengthening away from the crown of your head. Feel your hips open and your weight evenly releasing through your hips and pubic bone into the mat. Try to release your lower spine into its natural curve.

Check your ribcage: if you feel you are 'sitting' on the bottom of your ribs, lift your chest and tuck your ribcage under you to connect the front of your ribcage to your centre and allow your spine to lengthen. Release your ribs heavily into the mat.

Allow your shoulders to feel open and relaxed along your back, and the collarbones to be wide at the front. Soften your face and let your neck be free and in its natural curve.

Deepen the abdominal connection, and imagine you are gently lifting your lower abdominals away from the mat. Feel this soft engagement internally only: you should avoid gripping your buttocks or allowing your spine to move or become tense.

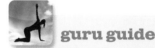 **guru guide**

• It is harder without the feedback of the floor underneath your back to determine whether your spine and pelvis are in neutral, so concentrate on the relationship between your pelvis, spine and ribcage.

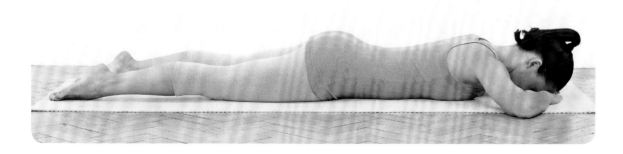

Cobra PREPARATION

◆ GOOD FOR: Spinal mobility, challenging muscles

This is a preparation for the classical exercise cobra, a wonderful way of mobilizing your spine in extension, requiring sequential control of your spine and working the deep abdominals.

guru guide

• Imagine your spine lengthening as you move. Move sequentially through your spine: head first, then neck, then chest.

• Allow your chest to stay open, and keep a soft pressure through your arms. Do not press too hard.

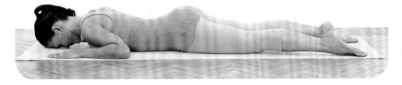

1 Align yourself centrally on your front, spine and pelvis in neutral (see page 25). Rest your forehead on the mat, bend your elbows and place your hands slightly wider than your shoulders, with your thumbs in line with your nose, palms facing down. Release the back of your shoulders and feel wide across your collarbones. Lengthen your legs straight, slightly wider than hip-width apart, and turned out from your hip. Gently engage your centre.

Repeat up to **10** times.

Related exercises

Cobra (page 104)

Swan dive (pages 128–9)

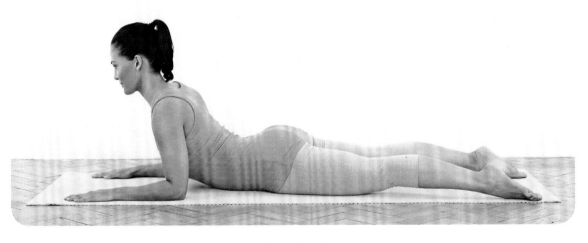

2 Breathe in to prepare and lengthen through your spine. Breathe out and begin to open the front of your neck as you roll your nose forward and up, lifting your chest off the mat. Keep your lower ribs in contact with the mat, but imagine you are opening your heart forward. Relax your shoulder blades. Breathe in to hold the position, keeping your abdominals lifted. Breathe out, and release your chest and head, returning to the start position. Repeat up to 10 times.

Rest position

◆ GOOD FOR: Warming up, cooling down

A yoga position known as 'child's pose', this relaxing exercise lengthens your spine, encouraging release of tension and deep wide breathing into your ribcage. Keep your knees together for more stretch in the lower back, or release your knees for more of a stretch in the inner thighs.

Start in four-point kneeling (see page 40). Bring your feet together, take a deep breath in and release your bottom towards your heels, opening your knees slightly if necessary. Allow your tailbone to soften and release your forehead towards the floor. Let your shoulders relax as your arms lengthen away from your body. Feel your weight releasing down to the floor.

Maintain a sense of connection and lift in your abdominals: this is not a position of collapse. Breathe in deeply through your nose, channelling your breath into the back of your body and feel your ribcage expand. Breathe out and allow your spine to release further into the position. Repeat for up to 10 breaths in this position.

To come out of this position: on an exhalation, draw in your abdominals and uncurl your spine. Drop your tailbone onto your heels and restack your spine to a sitting position.

guru guide

• If you have any knee problems, be careful with this position.

• If your lower back is very tight and there is a big space between your bottom and heels, place a cushion on your heels andencourage your bottom to release onto the cushion.

• Once you are in the rest position and breathing in deeply, imagine the breath is releasing deeply into the back of your body and that it is inflating every vertebra of your spine, down to your tailbone.

Breathe in deeply for up to 10 breaths.

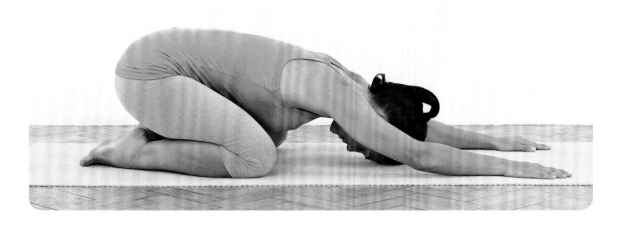

C-curve

◆ GOOD FOR: Warming up, spinal mobility, challenging muscles

This teaches you awareness of the c-curve alignment of your spine, using your abdominals to move sequentially bone by bone. It is needed for a number of exercises in this book. It challenges you to scoop your abdominals deeply without affecting the position of your spine.

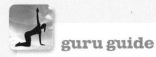

guru guide

• Make sure your abdominals are lifted and this is a lengthened position – do not collapse forward; think of lifting your ribcage away from your hips.

• Do not drop your head: keep it evenly flexed with the rest of your spine.

• Keep your neck long and do not hunch your shoulders.

• Move evenly and sequentially through your spine as you curl.

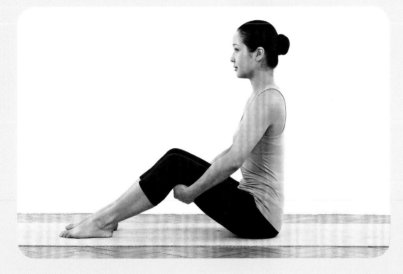

1 Sitting upright, bend your knees with your feet flat on the floor, hip-width apart. Place your hands behind your thighs, with your elbows soft. Breathe in to prepare and lengthen through your spine.

Finding your c-curve is a fundamental Pilates skill, so practise this one a lot.

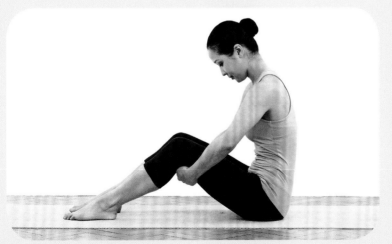

2 Tip your pelvis back by curling your tailbone underneath you and curl your lower spine sequentially. Nod your chin to your chest and curl your neck, head and upper back over your hips, creating a 'C' shape. Try to flex each part of your spine equally. The shoulders should be stacked above the hips. Keep your belly scooped as you round your spine, and feel long through both sides of the waist.

basic exercises **39**

Four-point kneeling

◆ GOOD FOR: Warming up, neutral spine and pelvis

This teaches you how to find your neutral spine and activate your deep stabilizing muscles, and to practise for exercises that start in a kneeling position.

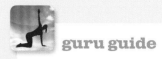

guru guide

• Do not allow your back to arch and dip the front of your body towards the floor – resist gravity with your muscles.

• Try not to disconnect your shoulder joints and hunch your shoulders. Relax your shoulder blades in towards your ribcage.

• Let your neck be long and your eye focus just above your fingertips on the mat.

• When practising Pilates breath, feel your shoulder blades relax into your back, and draw your arms into their sockets.

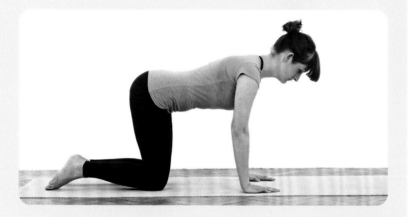

1 Kneel on all fours on the mat. Imagine your body is like a table, with your limbs as the legs, hands directly beneath your shoulders and knees directly beneath your hips. Make sure your elbows are not locked, and spread your weight evenly through your hands and along the front of your legs and feet.

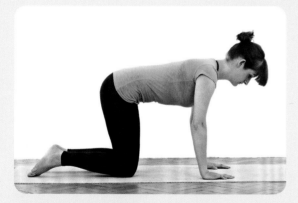

2 To find your neutral position, perform the pelvic tilts from page 27. Breathing normally throughout, engage your abdominals and gently curl your tailbone underneath you. Then lengthen your tailbone away from the crown of your head. Repeat this tilting movement a few times before settling in the centre.

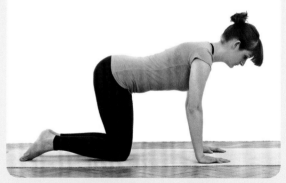

3 When your pelvis is centred, your hip and pubic bones should be level and your spine naturally curved. Now practise your Pilates breath. Breathe in to prepare and lengthen your spine. Breathe out and deeply engage your abdominals, lifting into the pelvic floor while keeping your spine long and still. Keep them scooped and breathe in widely into your ribcage. Build your strength by maintaining this position through a few full breaths.

Cat

◆ GOOD FOR: Warming up, spinal mobility, challenging muscles

This lovely exercise mobilizes the spine and works the abdominal muscles. It also encourages flowing movement and control.

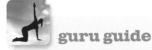

guru guide

• Make sure the flexion of your spine is even, with every part of it flexing to the same degree to create a c-curve.

• Try not to push up into your ribcage and ensure your neck does not collapse and drop your head in defeat: keep a natural line from your ribs through to the back of your head.

• COMMON MISTAKES TO AVOID (see below): when you return to neutral, try not to collapse your spine into an opposite arch and sink in the lower back. Instead, keep your spine long and in its natural curves.

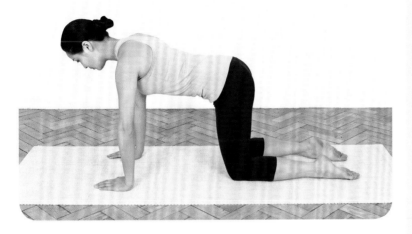

1 Start in the four-point kneeling position (see opposite). Find the neutral position of your spine: the natural curves should be present. Allow your tailbone to lengthen away from the crown of your head. Focus your eyes down towards the mat, just above your fingertips.

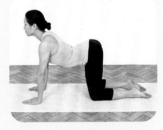

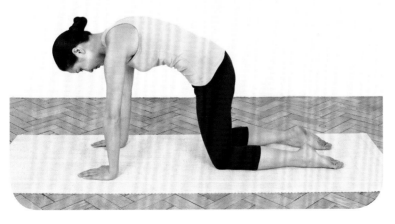

2 Breathe in wide into your ribcage, and feel your spine lengthen. Breathing out, draw your abdominals up and in, and begin to curl your tailbone underneath you. Curl your spine bone by bone into a c-curve. End by gently nodding your chin to your chest. Maintain the lift of your abdominals and an even weight through your hands and knees. Breathe in and, as you breathe out, unfurl your spine, releasing your tailbone away from the crown of your head to return to the neutral position. Repeat up to 10 times.

Repeat up to 10 times.

Standing correctly

◆ GOOD FOR: Warming up, cooling down

This teaches you an awareness of good posture,
encouraging you to settle your mind to your body, release
tension and feel how your body is connected as one unit.
Start by standing with bare feet on the floor.

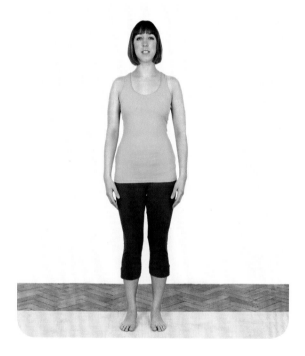 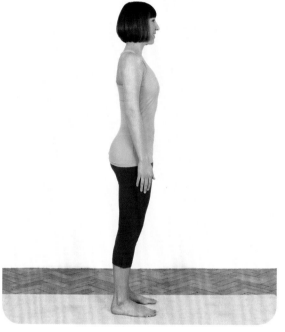

Position your feet beneath your hip joints,
feet in parallel. Relax your arms. Soften all ten
toes into the floor and feel heavy and even in
both feet. Soften your knees. Lengthen up
through the thighs and allow the hips to open.

Widen your collarbones across your front
and your shoulder blades in the back.

Feel your head balancing at the top of
your spine, lengthening the crown of your
head away from your feet. Keep your eye focus
forward and the muscles of your face relaxed.

Feel your pelvis in the neutral position,
tailbone lengthening to the floor.

Lengthen your waist, draw in your
stomach muscles and lift your pelvic floor.
Feel yourπ ribcage expand as you breathe in.
Imagine a straight line running from the top
of your head down to your ankles.

Stack your spine evenly and feel a
balance between your heels and toes. Allow
your arms to hang freely in their sockets with
your palms in line with your thighs.

Pilates stance

◆ GOOD FOR: Warming up, cooling down

This encourages you to become aware of your posture, activating your inner thigh and deep gluteal muscles. It is a position used in much of the advanced Pilates work, such as the hundred, stage 3 (see page 118).

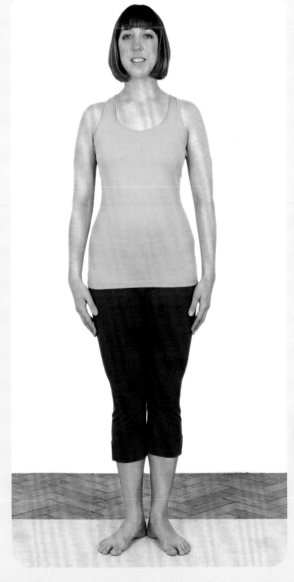

Standing correctly (see opposite), bring your heels together into a narrow V position: the size of a small slice of pizza in between your feet. Turn your entire leg out from your hip – feel your thighbone rotating within your hip joint. Relax your arms by the sides of your body and allow your chest to open and relax.

Release all ten toes down into the ground. Connect your heels and gently engage your inner thighs. Feel a lift in your buttocks. Lengthen your waist away from your pelvis, feeling the deep abdominal muscles.

Breathe and relax your facial muscles. Feel that you are grounded through your feet, but there is a lightness from the crown of your head, lengthening your spine to the ceiling.

guru guide

• Feel a sense of connection throughout your inner legs, from your heels up to your inner thighs.

• Avoid gripping and squeezing: it should feel like a gentle engagement of your inner thighs, buttocks and pelvic floor.

Rising on toes

◆ GOOD FOR: Warming up, joint mobility, cooling down

This exercise challenges your balance and teaches you good alignment of your feet, ankles, knees and hips.

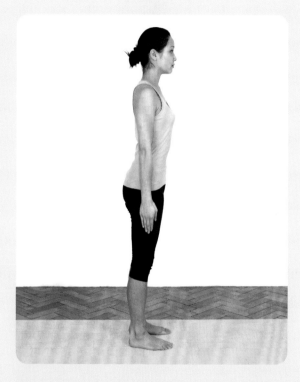

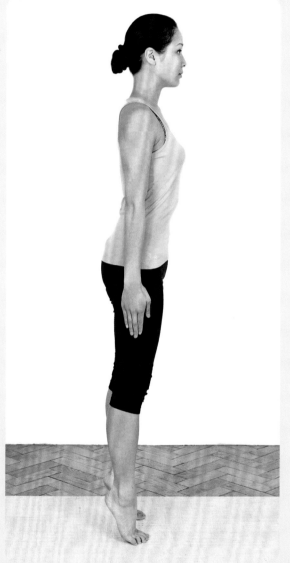

1 Standing correctly (see page 42), relax your arms by your sides and feel heavy and supported through your toes and heels. Engage your pelvic floor and draw in your abdominals. Soften your ribs and feel an even length in both sides of your waist.

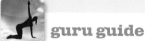 **guru guide**

• Maintain neutral spine throughout: ensure your back doesn't arch or flex forward as you rise up.

• Keep your toes connected to the ground: feel the weight evenly through the big and little toes.

• As a further challenge, try this with your eyes closed.

2 Breathe in to prepare and feel the length in your spine. As you breathe out, rise onto your toes. Breathe in and balance, maintaining a length through the body. Breathe out and lower your heels slowly to the floor: imagine your head stays lifted towards the ceiling. Soften your knees and, as you breathe in, return to the standing position. Repeat up to 10 times.

Floating arms

◆ GOOD FOR: Warming up, joint mobility, cooling down

This teaches you correct engagement of the muscles around your shoulders, encouraging smooth flowing movement of your arms around the shoulder joint.

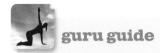
guru guide

• Keep your upper body open and weight even on both feet.

• Keep your abdominals engaged and ribs soft: make sure your upper body does not sway backwards.

Rising on toes + floating arms

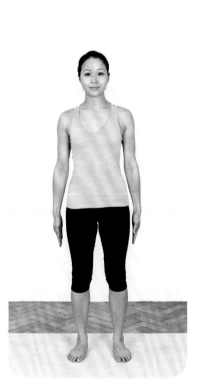

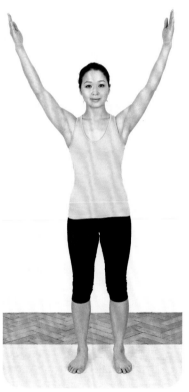

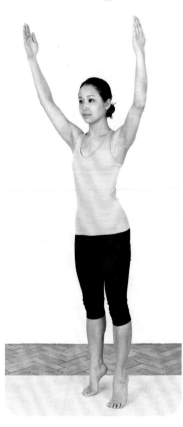

1 Standing correctly (see page 42), release your arms down by your sides and draw your abdominals in gently to lengthen your waist. Allow your neck to be free and relaxed. Soften your shoulders away from your ears. Feel grounded through your feet.

Repeat up to 5 times.

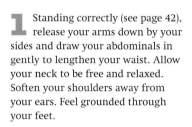

2 Breathe in to prepare and lengthen your spine. Then breathe out, engaging your abdominals as you raise your arms out by your sides. Imagine you have wings that are unfurling, with your arms soft at the elbow, palms open. Feel your shoulder blades opening on your back as you raise your arms. Your arms should be in your peripheral vision, not too far out to the side. Breathe in to lower the arms back down by your sides. Repeat up to 5 times.

1 As you begin to lift up onto your toes, simultaneously lengthen your arms above your head. Breathe in at the top and maintain the balance. Keep your eye focus forward and abdominals engaged. Breathe out, and release your heels slowly back to the floor, as you lower the arms down by your sides. Repeat 5 times.

Roll downs AGAINST THE WALL

◆ GOOD FOR: Warming up, spinal mobility, cooling down

This is a wonderful way to mobilize your spine, release tension in your shoulders, and strengthen your abdominals, back muscles, buttocks and legs.

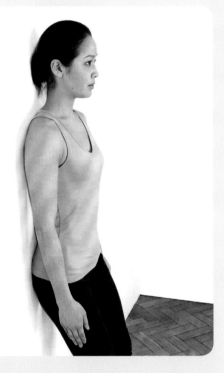

Repeat 5–10 times to warm up or cool down during a workout.

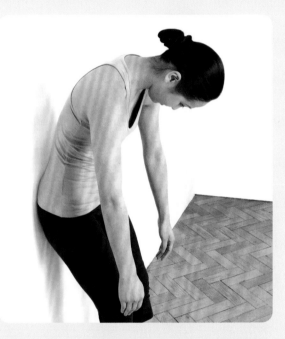

1 Stand tall with your feet hip-width apart and in parallel, with your back against a wall. Your feet should be about 30 cm (12 in) from the wall, with your knees soft. Your tailbone is heavy into the wall, pelvis and spine in neutral (see page 25). Soften your shoulders, and have your arms long and heavy by your sides.

guru guide

• Don't force your head back against the wall if it doesn't feel comfortable.

• Imagine your spine moving smoothly, rolling through each vertebra individually. Ensure every part of your spine is mobilized equally, like a wheel.

2 Breathe in, lengthen the back of your neck, look down your nose and nod your chin towards your chest. Breathe out as you roll your spine forward. Soften your breastbone and begin to peel your ribcage from the wall. Keep your abdominals lifted, hips still and allow your arms to soften and relax your shoulders and neck. Roll until you feel your tailbone about to move up the wall. Breathe in, keeping your abdominals strong. As you breathe out, begin to roll your pelvis underneath you, and wheel your spine back up against the wall using your abdominals, softening each vertebra individually and lengthening tall. Return your spine to neutral. Repeat 5–10 times.

Roll downs FREESTANDING

◆ GOOD FOR: Warming up, spinal mobility, cooling down

Freestanding roll downs require more balance and core strength than the wall version. The wall is no longer there for feedback, so you need to be aware of where your body is in space and carefully and gently control the movement with your core muscles.

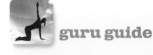

guru guide

• Do not attempt this exercise if you have a disc-related back problem.

• Keep your knees soft, and the weight even on both feet. Feel the weight equally over your toes and heels.

• Try to keep your breath flowing with the movement, breathing in to prepare to move, breathing out to move. Move slowly and evenly through your spine.

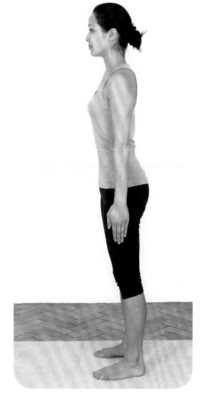

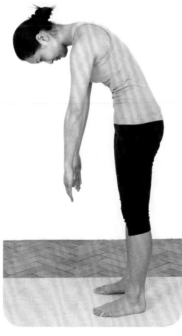

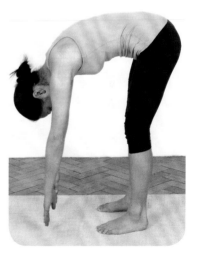

1 Stand with your feet hip-width apart and in parallel with soft knees and shoulders. Allow your arms to be heavy by your sides. Lengthen your spine to neutral (see page 25), imagine a heaviness around your tailbone. Draw in your abdominals throughout the exercise to support your spine.

2 Breathe in to lengthen the back of your neck, nodding your eyes and chin down. Breathe out and follow the roll down through your neck and ribcage, softening the front of your body as you lengthen through your back. Feel an openness through your lower back as the roll travels down your spine, bone by bone.

3 Keep your abdominals lifted and imagine you are hanging over a washing line, releasing down to gravity through your feet, arms and neck. Inhale and find the heaviness in your tailbone. As you breathe out, begin to roll your pelvis underneath you, and wheel your spine back up to neutral. Repeat 5–10 times.

Side reach

◆ GOOD FOR: Warming up, spinal mobility, stretching

This is a great way to stretch your waist and encourage correct and graceful shoulder movement, keeping your spine long and stable. It challenges the oblique muscles and can be performed standing or kneeling.

Repeat up to 5 times on both sides.

Side reach: kneeling

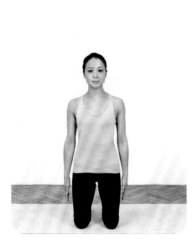 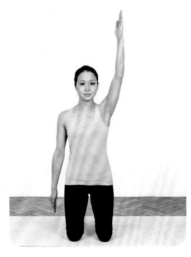 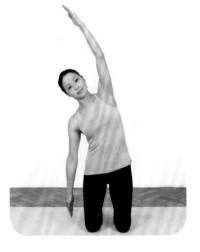

1 In an upright kneeling position, place your knees hip-width apart and elongate your spine into neutral. Lengthen your neck, draw in your abdominals and release your arms by your sides.

2 Breathe in wide and full and float your left arm out by your side and up to the ceiling. Keep your elbow soft and palm open.

3 As you breathe out, draw in your abdominals and lengthen the spine upwards as you reach the spine across to the side. Your arm naturally follows the movement, but do not lead with your arm. Feel your ribcage lengthen away from your pelvis. Feel grounded evenly through both knees and feel the stretch in the left side of your body. Breathe into the stretch, continuing to lengthen your torso. Allow your right arm to be relaxed down by your side. Breathe out and, keeping your abdominals strong, return your torso to the centre with control. Float your arm out by your side back to the start position. Repeat up to 5 times on both sides.

 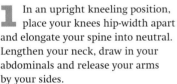 **guru guide**

• COMMON MISTAKES TO AVOID (see right): maintain a space between your shoulder and ear and keep your neck long. As you reach across to the side try to avoid twisting your torso and hips, and collapsing the waist. Keep your hips square and waist long on both sides.

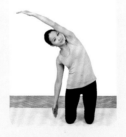

Side reach: standing

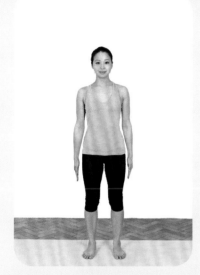

1 Standing correctly (see page 42), relax your arms and allow the spine to release into neutral (see page 25). Engage your pelvic floor, draw in your abdominals and soften your ribs.

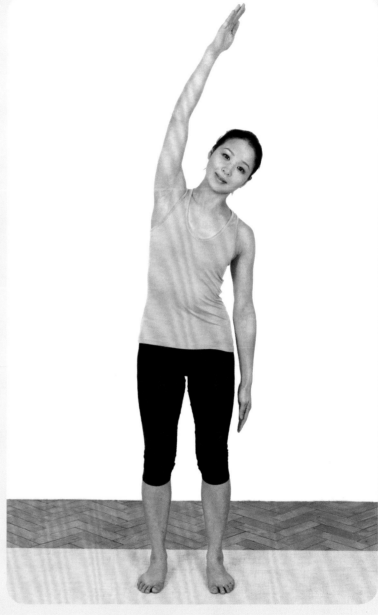

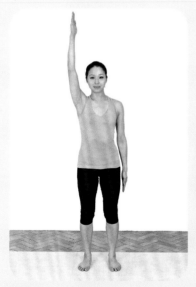

2 Breathe in wide and full and float your left arm out by your side and up to the ceiling. Keep your elbow soft and palm open.

3 Breathe out and lengthen your spine diagonally. Feel the stretch along your side and feel grounded evenly through both feet, trying not to sway your body to the side. Allow your other arm to fall naturally by your side. Keep both sides of your waist long. Keep your eye focus forward, imagine you are bending between two panes of glass and avoid rotating your body forward or back. Breathe out and, keeping your abdominals strong, return your torso to the centre with control. Float your arm out by your side, back to the start position. Repeat up to 5 times on both sides.

Waist twist

◆ GOOD FOR: Warming up, spinal mobility, cooling down

This teaches you how to rotate your spine with stability and length. It challenges your abdominal muscles and encourages an awareness of your posture.

For **each exercise repeat 5 times** to **either side**.

Waist twist: sitting

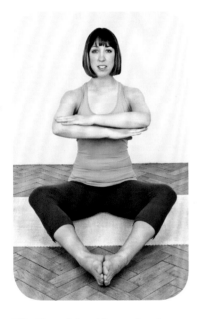

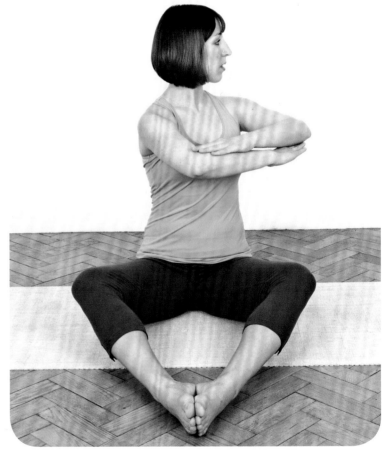

1 Sit upright with your legs bent in front of you and the soles of your feet connected. Sit directly on your sitting bones, with your spine and pelvis in neutral (see page 25). If you need to, sit on a folded towel or a cushion to make sure your spine is in neutral. Fold your arms in front of you, level with your breastbone. Deepen your abdominals, grow tall and feel your waist lifting away from your pelvis.

2 Breathe in to prepare and lengthen the spine. Breathe out, and rotate your torso to the left. Keep your hips facing forward and try not to allow your pelvis to rotate with the spine. Breathe in, continue to lengthen your spine and keep your abdominals strong as you return to the start position. Breathe out and twist to the opposite side. Make sure your arms stay square to the torso and feel the deep abdominals initiating and supporting the twist. Repeat 5 times to each side.

Waist twist: standing

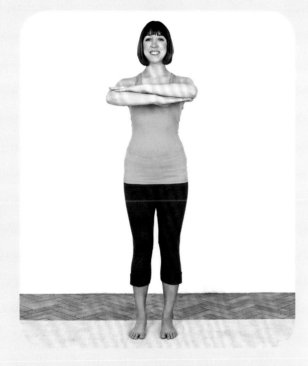

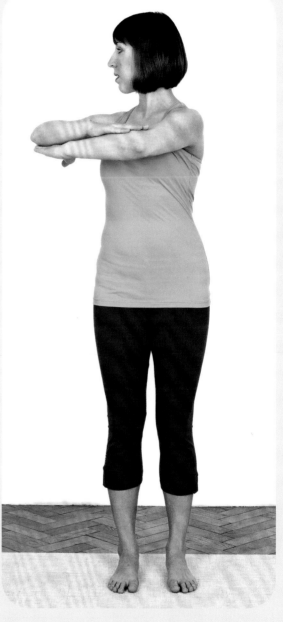

1 Standing correctly (see page 42) and with your spine in neutral (see page 25), fold your arms in front of your chest, level with your breastbone.

guru guide

• COMMON MISTAKES TO AVOID (see right): make sure the movement comes from your spine and abdominals, not from leading with your elbows. Maintain the arms' shape throughout and keep your hips square.

• Keep lifting up through the crown of your head to avoid tilting your spine and arching back. Imagine growing taller as you twist.

• If it is more comfortable, do the sitting waist twist in a chair with your feet hip-width apart on the floor.

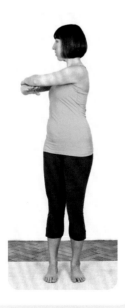

2 Breathe in to prepare and lengthen your spine. As you breathe out, twist your torso to the right. Be careful to ensure your hips do not twist with your spine. Keep your abdominals strong. Breathe in and maintain the length of your spine as you return to the starting position. As you breathe out, twist in the opposite direction. Repeat 5 times.

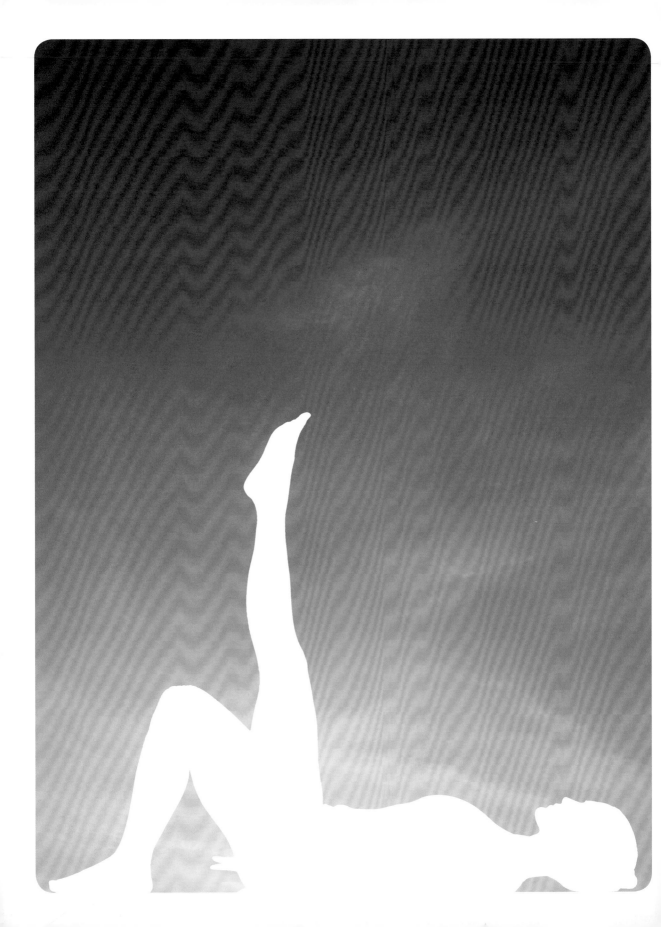

Beginner exercises

In this section you move on from the basics and add to the challenge and level of skill required. As with the basics, the exercises are suitable for anyone who is new to Pilates, and can also serve as a reminder for those wanting to add to their practice. They can be seen as a stepping stone to the more advanced work, but should be continually revisited and are valuable for balancing your body and providing strength and release, however advanced you are.

Starfish

◆ GOOD FOR: Warming up, joint mobility, cooling down

This challenges you to maintain a stable pelvis and spine as you move your limbs independently from a strong centre, with flow and control. It also challenges your coordination. It combines the principles seen in leg slides (see page 28) and ribcage closure (see page 30).

Related exercises

Leg slides (page 28)

Ribcage closure (page 30)

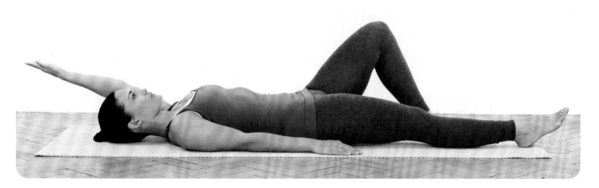

1 Align yourself in the relaxation position. Breathe in to prepare and lengthen your spine. Breathe out, engage your pelvic floor and scoop your lower abdominals, as you reach one arm up and back towards the floor. Simultaneously, lengthen your opposite leg in line with your hip. Do not allow your ribcage to arch. Breathe in as you lengthen your limbs away from your centre, and breathe out to return them back to the start position. Repeat up to 10 times on each side.

guru guide

• Only reach your arm as far as you can maintain neutral spine.

• Stay grounded and still through your supporting leg. Draw your leg back using the muscles of the back of your thigh and buttock rather than gripping the front of your thigh.

Making it harder

To vary the pace of the exercise as you become more confident with it, breathe out to lengthen your limbs, and breathe in to return.

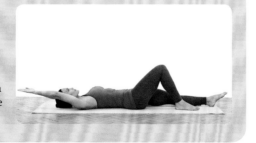

Repeat up to 10 times on each side.

Shoulder drops

◆ GOOD FOR: Warming up, joint mobility, cooling down

This is a great way of releasing tension and relaxing your shoulder and neck area, encouraging you to become aware of the relationship of your arms to your torso and the range of movement in your shoulder joint.

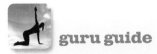

guru guide

• Do not allow your body to rock as you reach each arm. It is a movement just of your shoulder blade, and your pelvis and spine should stay stable.

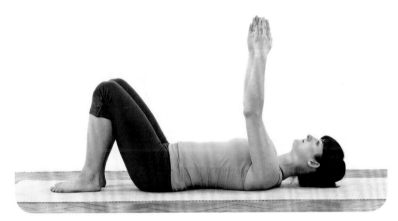

Repeat up to 10 times on each arm.

1 Align yourself in the relaxation position. Raise both arms up towards the ceiling in line with your shoulders, palms facing each other. Relax the back of your shoulders and engage your centre at a low level throughout this exercise.

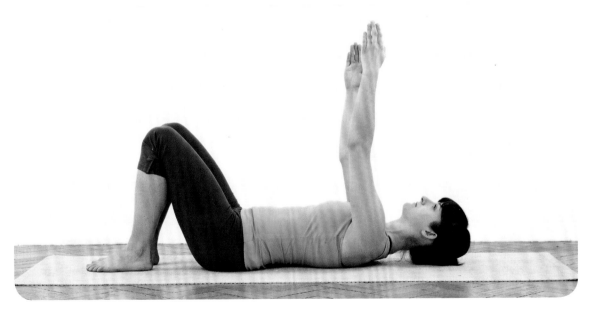

2 Breathe in to reach one arm up towards the ceiling, feeling your shoulder blade peel off the mat and releasing from your ribcage. Breathe out to release your arm back down, drawing it softly back into its socket and feel your shoulder blade drop into the mat once more. Repeat up to 10 times on each arm.

Curl ups

◆ GOOD FOR: Spinal mobility, challenging muscles

The basic curl up is a fantastic way of strengthening the abdominals, mobilizing the spine while maintaining neutral pelvis. The curl up with single knee fold adds further challenge to the stability of your pelvis and abdominal strength.

Repeat the basic curl up up to **10 times.**

Basic curl up

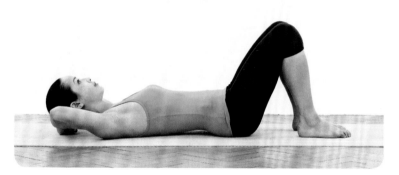

1 Start in the relaxation position, pelvis and spine in neutral. Clasp your hands together behind your head, releasing your elbows wide but keeping them in your peripheral vision. Keep your shoulders relaxed and away from your ears and neck long. Allow your head to be heavy in your hands.

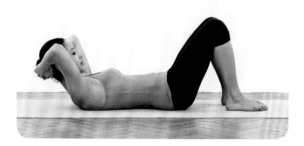

2 Breathe in to prepare and lengthen your spine. As you breathe out, engage your pelvic floor and deep abdominals, lengthen the back of your neck and nod your chin to your chest to begin to curl your spine off the mat. Curl your spine as far as you can maintain neutral pelvis. Keep your pelvis still, abdominals scooped and eye focus towards your navel.

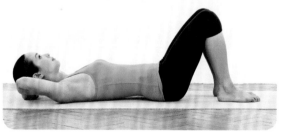

3 Breathe in to maintain this position and, as you breathe out, lower slowly back down with control, keeping your abdominal muscles working. Keep your elbows in your peripheral vision throughout. Try not to lose the connection with your shoulder joints and let them 'pop' open when you reach the mat. Repeat up to 10 times.

Curl ups with single knee fold

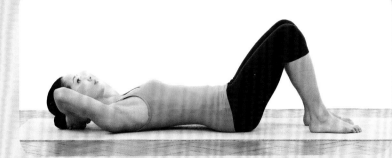

guru guide

• As you curl up, imagine you have a piece of tape running from your breastbone to your pubic bone. Make sure you keep the tape from wrinkling by allowing your torso to stay long.

• Once you are familiar with the curl up, you may alter your breath: breathe out to curl up, breathe in to curl down.

• Make sure you keep the neutral position of your pelvis. Curl up only as far as you can while keeping the pelvis still.

• COMMON MISTAKES TO AVOID (see below): don't lead the movement with your elbows and hug your head. Instead, keep your elbows wide and in your peripheral vision. Keep your head heavy and neck long. If you are doing a curl up with a single knee fold, as you float your knee in, make sure you don't lose neutral by dropping your lower back into the mat and collapsing your knee into your chest.

1 Start in the relaxation position, as for step 1, opposite. Breathe in to prepare and lengthen your spine.

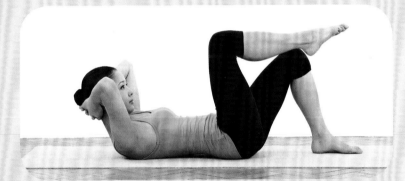

2 As you breathe out, nod your chin to your chest and use your abdominals to begin to curl your spine off the mat. Simultaneously float your right knee in towards your chest, maintaining neutral pelvis – use your abdominals to ensure your lower spine does not imprint into the mat. Keep your tailbone heavy.

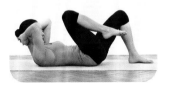

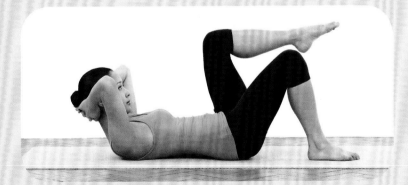

3 Breathe in and float your knee down as you simultaneously return your head and shoulders to the mat, with control. Repeat for the other leg. Repeat up to 5 times on each leg.

Repeat up to 5 times on each leg.

Obliques

◆ GOOD FOR: Spinal mobility, challenging muscles

These exercises challenge your abdominal and waist muscles, requiring you to control your spinal movement while maintaining neutral pelvis.

guru guide

• For obliques with leg slide, imagine a piece of string tied from your nose to your big toe, and coordinate your torso and leg movement to the same timing.

• COMMON MISTAKES TO AVOID (see below): keep your elbows wide and head heavy. Make sure the movement comes from your ribcage and abdominals, not from your elbows. Imagine funnelling your ribcage across to one hip and then the other. Ensure it is just the ribcage that rotates: your pelvis should stay heavy and grounded, and your body should not tip over to one side.

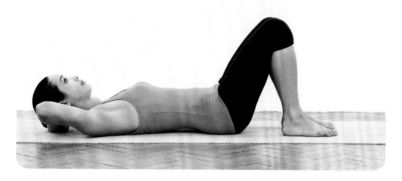

1 Begin in the relaxation position, pelvis and spine in neutral. Clasp your hands together behind your head, releasing your elbows wide but keeping them in your peripheral vision. Keep your shoulders relaxed and away from your ears and keep your neck long. Allow your head to be heavy in your hands.

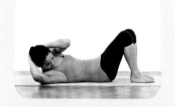

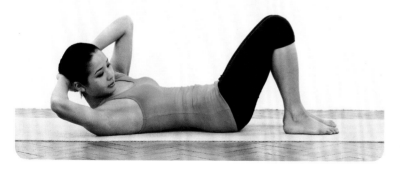

Repeat up to **10 times** on each side.

2 Breathe in to prepare and lengthen your spine. Breathe out as you nod your chin towards your chest, and begin to curl your upper body off the mat. Rotate your spine to the right, directing your breastbone towards your right hip. Feel your waist and lower abdominal muscles working. Keep your feet grounded and pelvis still – twist only from your ribs. Breathe in wide into your ribcage and maintain the position, deepening your abdominal connection. Breathe out and slowly release to the centre. Repeat up to 10 times on each side.

Related exercise

Criss cross (pages 140–1)

Obliques with leg slide

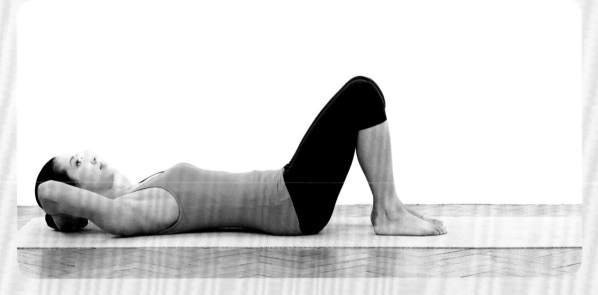

1 Start in the relaxation position, as for step 1, opposite. Breathe in to prepare and lengthen your spine.

Breathe out as you nod your chin towards your chest and begin to curl your upper body off the mat.

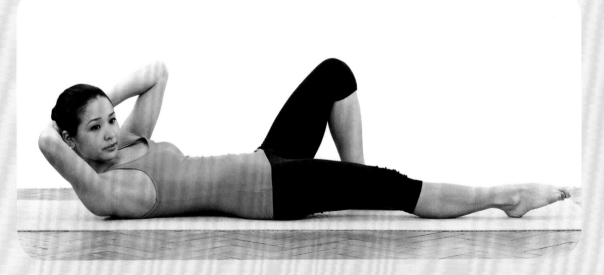

2 At the same time, begin to lengthen your right leg along the floor directly in line with your body. Rotate your spine to the right, directing your breastbone towards your right hip, and continue the posture as for step 2,

opposite. To change legs, breathe out and gently draw your right leg back towards your bottom as you release your head and shoulders back to centre ready to make an oblique with leg slide on the other side. Repeat up to 10 times on each side.

Hip rolls: feet down

◆ GOOD FOR: Warming up, spinal mobility

This challenges the abdominals and obliques, and requires the ability to mobilize your spine with control, maintaining softness and release in your upper body.

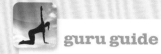

guru guide

• Keep your abdominals strong and make sure your back does not arch: connect your ribcage towards your hips to keep a length in your torso.

• Control the movement of your legs with your abdominals: try not to allow them to drop heavily to the side.

• Make sure your legs stay connected from your inner thighs to your big toes. If it helps, place a cushion between your knees.

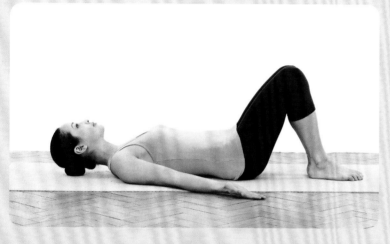

1 Start in the relaxation position. Bring your feet and knees together with a strong connection with your inner thighs and engage your pelvic floor. Relax your shoulders and release your arms slightly wider than your sides, palms facing up or down, whichever feels more stable for you.

Related exercise

Hip rolls: feet up (page 61)

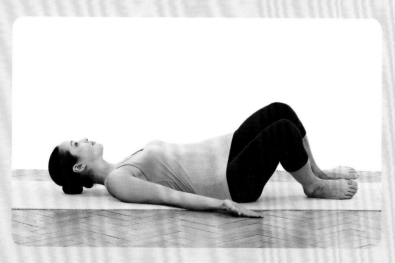

2 Breathe in to prepare and lengthen through your spine. Engage your centre as you begin to rotate your hips and legs to the right. Keep your knees connected. Stay heavy across your shoulders and keep your eye focus directly towards the ceiling. The left side of your bottom and pelvis will peel slightly from the mat. Allow your foot to naturally follow the movement: the soles of your feet will peel off the mat also. Breathe out and deepen your abdominals to return your pelvis and legs back to the start position. Breathe in at the centre and roll to the other side. Repeat up to 5 times on each side.

Repeat up to 5 times on each side.

Hip rolls: feet up

◆ GOOD FOR: Warming up, spinal mobility, challenging muscles

This is a greater challenge for the abdominals and obliques. A strong centre is required to control the spinal movement, maintaining release in your upper body.

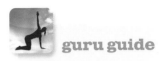

guru guide

• Make sure your back does not arch: connect your ribcage towards your hips to keep a length in your torso.

• Stay heavy and grounded across your shoulder blades and allow your arms to support your movement.

• Make sure your legs stay connected. Try not to allow your knees to break apart as you roll, they should stay level and connected – if it helps, place a cushion between your knees.

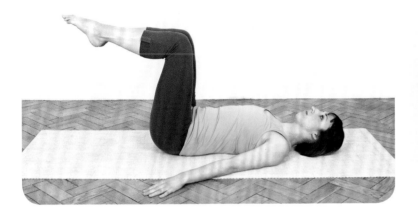

1 Starting in the relaxation position, float one knee and then the other into a double knee fold (see page 35). Draw your feet and knees together, ensure a strong connection with your inner thighs and engage your pelvic floor. Relax your shoulders and release your arms out slightly wider than your sides, palms facing up or down, whichever feels more stable for you.

Related exercise

Hip rolls: feet down (page 60)

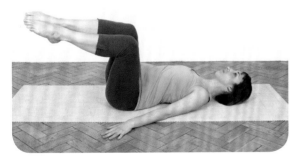

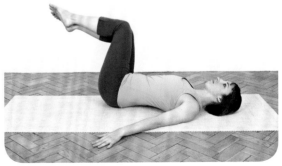

2 Breathe in to prepare and lengthen through your spine. Deepen the abdominal connection as you begin to rotate your hips and legs to the left. Keep your shoulders wide and heavy, and eye focus directly towards the ceiling. The right side of your bottom and pelvis will peel slightly from the mat.

3 Breathe out and deepen your abdominals to return your pelvis and legs back to the start position. Breathe in at the centre, and roll to the other side. Repeat up to 5 times on each side.

Hamstring stretch

◆ GOOD FOR: Warming up, stretching, cooling down

This is a great way to stretch the hamstring muscles at the back of your thigh, while you maintain a stable and relaxed torso.

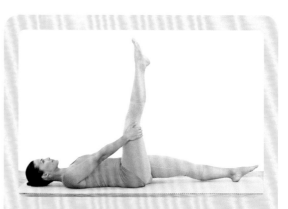

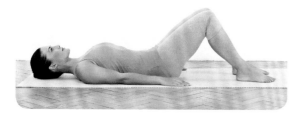

1 Align yourself in the relaxation position, with one or two small cushions underneath your head if needed, to enable your shoulders to relax.

Making it harder

If you feel stable with your supporting foot grounded, you can add challenge to this stretch by lengthening your supporting leg along the floor. This requires more core stability in order to control your torso as you lengthen your leg.

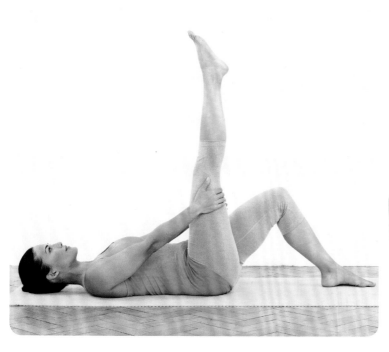

2 Breathe in wide to prepare and lengthen your spine. Breathe out, engage your centre and float one leg towards you. Place your hands around the back of your thigh to draw your knee slightly towards you, and release your leg up towards the ceiling. Feel your tailbone anchored and heavy into the floor. Breathe normally, relax your shoulders and spine, and keep your pelvis in neutral as you feel the stretch. After a few breaths, return to the relaxation position. Repeat on the other side.

 guru guide

• Only straighten your leg as far as you feel comfortable – it should be a stretch not a strain.

• Stay open in the chest with your collarbones wide and elbows soft.

Hip flexor stretch

◆ GOOD FOR: Warming up, stretching, cooling down

This is a wonderful way to release the front of your hip and gently stretch your hip flexors. It is important to balance these muscles if you sit at a desk all day or drive a lot, as they are held permanently in a shortened position.

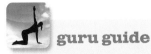

guru guide

• Stay soft and relaxed in your neck, jaw and shoulders, and keep your elbows open.

• If it is more comfortable, place your hands around the back of your thigh to draw your knee in.

• Keep your upper body relaxed but abdominals strong.

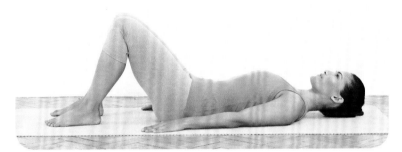

1 Align yourself in the relaxation position, with one or two small cushions underneath your head if needed, to enable your shoulders to relax.

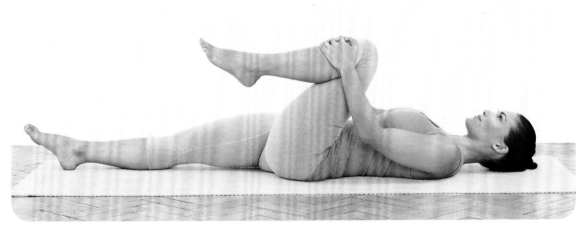

2 Breathe in wide to prepare and lengthen your spine. Breathe out, engage your centre and float one leg in towards you, dropping your thighbone into its joint. Place your hands around the front of the knee to draw it towards your chest. Breathe in and, as you breathe out, slide the other leg away in line with your body. Maintain neutral pelvis and spine. Feel a heaviness in the extended leg to try to gently release the front of your hip. Breathe into the stretch for several breaths and then, on an out breath, return your extended leg to the start position, and float the knee down. Repeat on the other side.

The hundred PREPARATION

◆ GOOD FOR: Warming up

The hundred is one of the classical Pilates exercises. It is often used as a warm-up in some schools of Pilates, and once you've practised it, you will understand why. This preparation teaches you how to find the deep lateral Pilates breath while working the abdominals and coordinating the arm beats. The hundred utilizes every principle of Pilates beautifully. Start with the preparation and first stage for this exercise (opposite), and when you feel you have mastered it, move on to the intermediate and advanced stages on pages 88 and 118.

guru guide

• If you lose the abdominal scoop as you breathe in, practise until you can maintain it.

• Keep your neck relaxed as you beat. Isolate the movement of your arms from your torso.

• Try to keep your breath soft, don't puff or pant the air out of your lips in time with the beating.

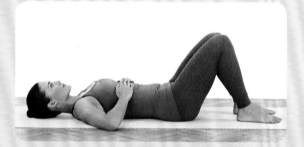

1 Lie in the relaxation position with your hands on your lower ribcage. Breathe in and feel your ribcage open. Breathe out, feel it close as you deepen your abdominals, lift your pelvic floor and scoop your belly. Breathe in and try to maintain this scoop. Practise with up to 10 breaths.

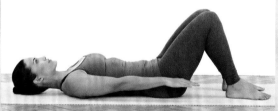

2 To practise the hundred arm beats with the breath, extend your arms by your sides. Lengthen your arms above the ground, through to your fingertips, and breathe in deeply.

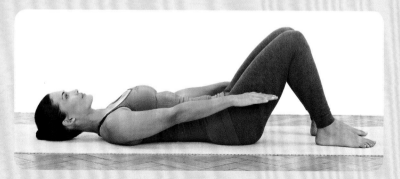

3 As you breathe in, pump up and down for a count of 5, beating up to mid-thigh height. Keep your shoulders relaxed, moving your arms from the joint. Breathe out and beat for another count of 5. Repeat this 20 times to make up to 100 beats.

Related exercises

The hundred: stages 1, 2 and 3 (pages 65, 88 and 118)

Beat your arms 100 times.

The hundred STAGE 1

◆ GOOD FOR: Challenging muscles, spinal mobility

Following on from the hundred preparation, opposite, learn how to coordinate deep abdominal work with the breath and the arm beats. Stage 1 needs core control, so master it before progressing to stage 2 on page 88.

Related exercises

The hundred preparation and stages 2 and 3 (pages 64, 88 and 118)

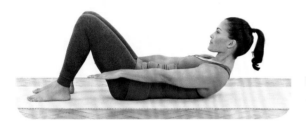

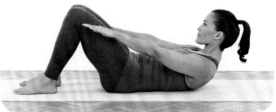

1 Lie in the relaxation position. Breathe in wide and full to prepare. As you breathe out, engage your centre, nod your chin to your chest and curl your upper body off the mat. Simultaneously lengthen your arms above the floor by your sides.

2 Keeping your abdominals scooped, breathe in and beat your arms for a count of 5. Breathe out and beat for a count of 5, up to a count of 100. Release your upper body down to the mat on an out breath. Finish with some neck rolls (see page 33) to release any tension around your neck.

guru guide

• If you feel breathless or lightheaded, stop at once.

• Keep your upper body open, your shoulder blades wide and down, and your neck relaxed.

• Make sure the beating movement is just in your arms and not in your torso.

• COMMON MISTAKES TO AVOID (see below): never allow your eye focus to be up to the ceiling or you will unnecessarily strain your neck. Focus your eyes towards your navel and keep your abdominals scooped deeply.

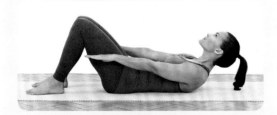

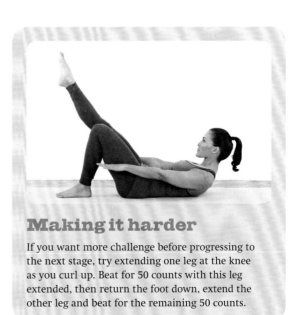

Making it harder

If you want more challenge before progressing to the next stage, try extending one leg at the knee as you curl up. Beat for 50 counts with this leg extended, then return the foot down, extend the other leg and beat for the remaining 50 counts.

Single leg stretch STAGE 1

◆ GOOD FOR: Challenging muscles, stretching

Another exercise from the classical mat repertoire, the advanced single leg stretch is a highly effective abdominal workout in itself, combining all Pilates principles. Stage 1 teaches you to coordinate your breath with the movement of your limbs from a strong centre, moving smoothly with precision. Once this is easy and the hand patterning feels automatic, progress to stage 2.

Repeat up to 10 times.

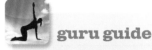

guru guide

• Keep your leg pointing directly up to the ceiling; do not allow it to fall towards the floor.

Related exercises

Single leg stretch: stages 2 and 3 (pages 92–3 and 119)

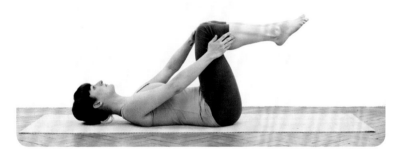

1 Lie in the relaxation position with your pelvis and spine in neutral. Breathe in wide and full to prepare. As you breathe out, gently engage your centre and double knee fold your legs towards your chest. Keep your back anchored to the floor throughout.

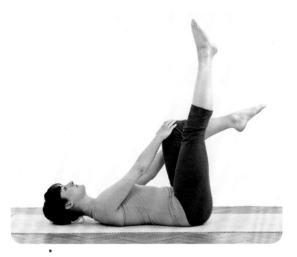

2 Breathe in and take your left hand across the left knee. Extend your right hand down the side of your shin. Breathe out, deepen your abdominals and straighten your right leg directly to the ceiling.

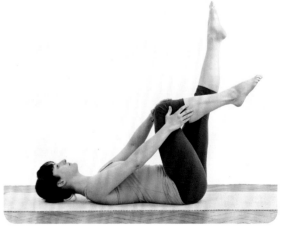

3 Breathe in, and bend your right knee back towards your chest and change your hand position onto the left knee. Breathe out and extend your left leg. Repeat up to 10 times on each leg.

Double leg stretch STAGE 1

◆ GOOD FOR: Challenging muscles, stretching

This exercise strengthens your abdominals and leg muscles, focusing on stamina, smooth movement, coordination and control. This is another advanced mat exercise, broken down into stages so you will be fully prepared for the classical version on pages 120–1.

Related exercise

Double leg stretch: stage 2 (pages 120–1)

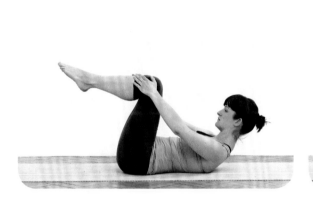

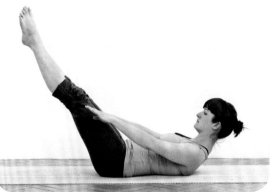

1 Lie in the relaxation position with your pelvis and spine in neutral. Breathe in wide and full to prepare. As you breathe out, gently engage your centre and double knee fold your legs (see page 35). Have your feet and knees together and place your hands lightly around your knees. Breathe out, engage your core and nod your chin to your chest to curl your upper body off the mat. Breathe in to prepare and lengthen your spine.

2 Breathe out, deepen your abdominals and press your legs away from your centre, towards the ceiling. Keep your legs in parallel, with your inner thighs engaged and toes softly pointed. Simultaneously, release your arms forward above the floor, about mid-thigh height. Breathe in and fold your knees back towards your chest as you release your upper body down towards the mat. Repeat up to 10 times.

guru guide

• Keep your legs high and ensure your abdominals are scooped strongly to keep your pelvis in neutral.

• Keep your eye focus towards your thighs.

Repeat up to 10 times on each leg.

Making it easier

If you feel a strain in your neck, interlace your hands behind your head and support its weight as you lengthen your legs away from you in step 2.

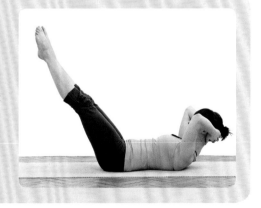

Knee circles

◆ GOOD FOR: Warming up, joint mobility

This exercise teaches you to move your thighbone independently of the pelvis, which helps to mobilize your hip joint. Concentrate throughout on the precision of your movement.

Related exercises

Leg circles: stages 1 and 2
(pages 69 and 90–1)

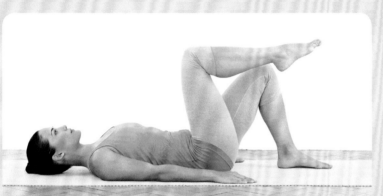

 guru guide

• Imagine the movement coming from your thighbone circling in the socket, not leading with your foot or knee. The knee joint angle remains the same throughout. Think of your thighbone as being like a spoon turning in a glass.

Repeat 8 times in each **direction** and with **each leg.**

1 Lie in the relaxation position with your pelvis and spine in neutral. Breathe in to prepare. As you breathe out, gently engage your centre and float one knee in towards your chest. Breathing with the movement, begin to circle your thighbone towards your centre.

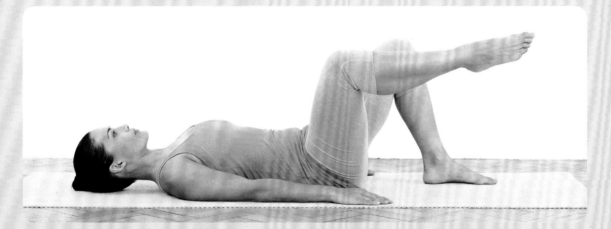

2 Continue to circle around, down and back up to the start position. Find a full range of movement that does not disturb the neutral position of your pelvis. Repeat up to 8 times, then reverse the circles. Start with small circles and build up to larger movements, as long as you can keep your pelvis still. Float your leg back down to the start position, and repeat with the other leg.

Leg circles STAGE 1

◆ GOOD FOR: Joint mobility, challenging muscles

This exercise adds greater challenge than the knee circles opposite. It takes more abdominal control to circle your leg freely from your hip while ensuring that you don't move your pelvis or torso.

Related exercises

Knee circles (page 68)

Leg circles: stage 2 (pages 90–1)

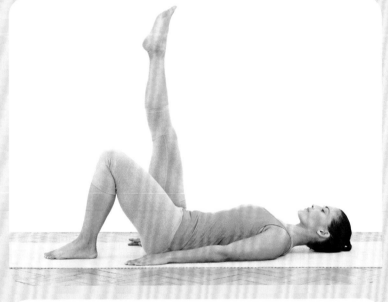

 guru guide

• Keep the supporting leg grounded and feel heavy through your tailbone.

• Maintain the slight turnout of the thighbone in its socket throughout the circle.

1 Lie in the relaxation position with your pelvis and spine in neutral. Breathe in to prepare. As you breathe out, engage your centre and float one knee in towards your chest. Breathing with the movement, straighten your leg towards the ceiling, turning the leg out slightly from the hip and keeping your knee soft.

Repeat 8 times in each direction and with each leg.

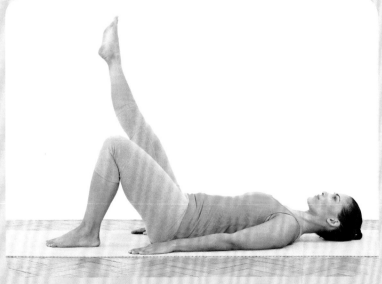

2 Begin to circle your thighbone towards your centre, and continue to circle around, down and back up to the start position. Be careful not to allow your pelvis to rock and there to be any movement in your torso at all. Repeat up to 8 times, then reverse the circles. Bend and float your leg back to the start position, and repeat with your other leg.

Roll backs

◆ GOOD FOR: Challenging muscles, spinal mobility

This is a tough exercise, great for toning the abdominals, and challenging the c-curve alignment of your spine.

Related exercise

C-curve (page 39)

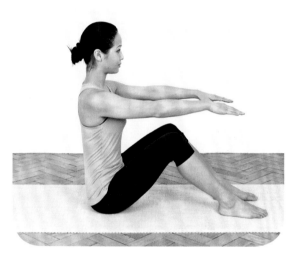

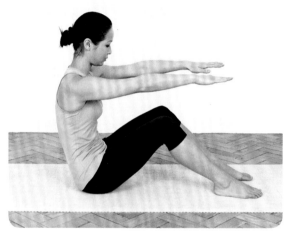

1 Sit upright, with your feet in line with your hips, parallel and grounded on the mat. Find your neutral position for the pelvis and spine, and feel your spine lengthening up. Reach your arms out in front of you, in line with your shoulders, palms facing down.

2 Breathe in and tilt your pelvis slightly to lengthen the spine into a c-curve, curving your shoulders directly over your hips. Make sure you do not collapse your shoulders forward, but feel long and lifted through the back of your head.

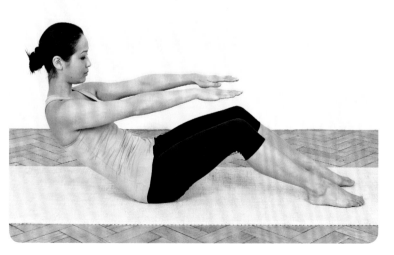

Breathe in to **maintain** this **position.**

3 Breathe out, roll your pelvis underneath you and release your spine back, until you can feel that your tailbone is supported by the mat. Breathe in to maintain this position. Keep your abdominals strong and feel your ribcage lifting away from your waist. Keep your fingertips lengthening forward.

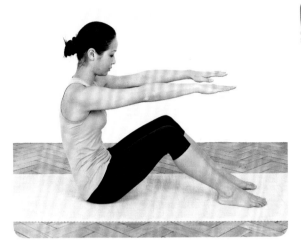

- Maintain an openness across your chest and the back of your shoulders.

- Try to move directly through the centre of your spine, not to one side more than the other.

- COMMON MISTAKES TO AVOID (see below): try not to allow your shoulders to hunch or your chest to collapse. Keep your neck long and released. Let your arms move naturally with your spine through the movement.

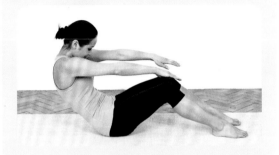

4 Breathe out as you roll forward, leading with the crown of your head. Imagine a lightness with the crown of your head lifting you back into the sitting position. Maintain the c-curve in your spine and keep your abdominals strong to restack your shoulders above your hips. Then, release your head back on top of your spine as you tilt your pelvis back into the neutral starting position.

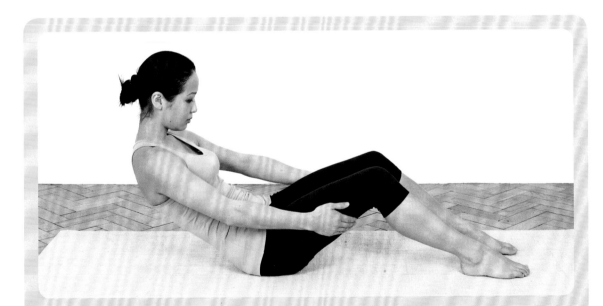

Making it easier

If your abdominals need assistance as they build strength, place your hands behind your thighs. As you move your spine back, allow your hands to travel down the back of your thigh, and as you restack the spine, let your hands move lightly back towards your knees. Do not grip or pull on your thighs, but allow your hands to guide and support you through the movement. Make sure your shoulders stay soft and away from your ears.

Table top

◆ GOOD FOR: Challenging muscles, joint mobility

This exercise challenges your ability to move your limbs from a strong stable centre, with control and balance. It is a great way of toning your abdominals by working against gravity and your own body weight.

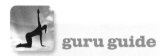

guru guide

• Imagine you are balancing a tray of drinks on your back: you don't want to dip on one side and allow the drinks to fall, so keep your belly working hard to stabilize the spine.

• Maintain a space between your shoulder and ear at all times.

• Keep your waist the same length on either side: do not allow your hip to hitch towards the shoulder as you move the leg.

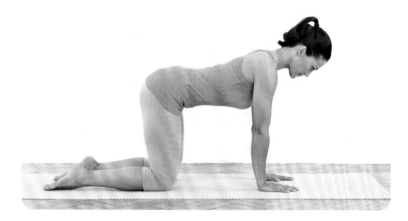

1 Align yourself in four-point kneeling (see page 40), with your hands directly beneath your shoulders and knees beneath your hips. Ensure your spine is in neutral, neck long and released and your eye focus is down into the mat, just above your hands.

Repeat 8 times with the opposite **arm and leg.**

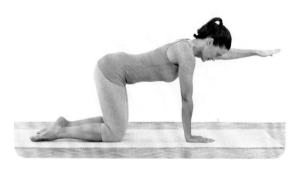

2 Breathe in to prepare and lengthen through your spine. Breathe out, draw in your abdominals and lengthen one arm forward, reaching in line with your shoulder. If this causes a strain around the shoulder and your spine moves, keep your arm lower. Breathe in to lower your arm, and repeat on the other side.

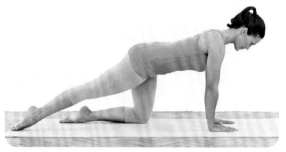

3 Breathe in to prepare and lengthen through your spine. Breathe out, deepen your connection to your centre and, maintaining your stable pelvis and spine, slide one leg behind you, in line with your body. Keep your foot softly pointed and in contact with the mat.

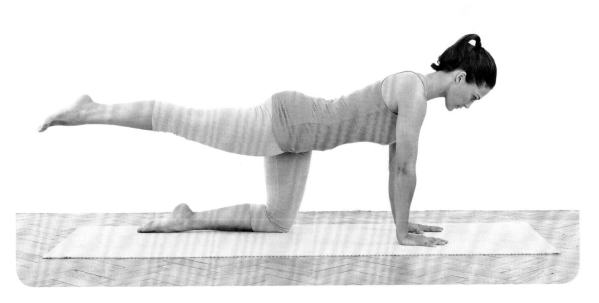

4 Breathe in to lengthen and lift your leg to hip height. Breathe out to lower your leg and then repeat on the other side. If you find that it is too challenging to raise your leg to hip height, keep your foot in contact with the floor until you have mastered balancing in this position.

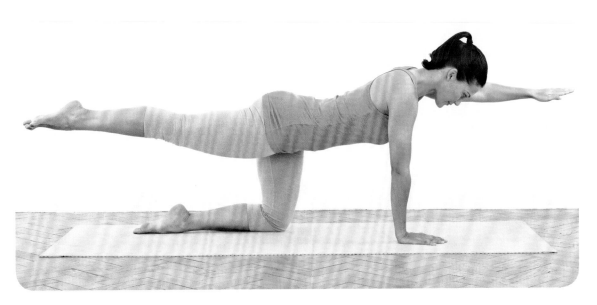

5 Breathe in to prepare and lengthen through your spine. Breathe out, deepen your connection to your centre and, maintaining your stable pelvis and spine, slide one leg behind you in line with your body, then raise it in line with your hips and, simultaneously, raise your opposite arm forward. Keep your eye focus down and neck long. Repeat with the opposite arm and leg 8 times.

Dart

◆ GOOD FOR: Spinal mobility, challenging muscles

This lovely exercise tones the muscles of the mid back, arms and inner thighs, mobilizing the upper spine. It is a wonderful way of counteracting poor posture by extending the spine and strengthening your back muscles.

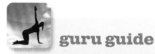

guru guide

• Keep your eye focus down towards the mat and your neck lengthened.

• COMMON MISTAKES TO AVOID (see below): try not to allow your legs to lift, keep them heavy and grounded. Feel a sense of length in your entire body, as if you are releasing the crown of your head away from your toes to touch opposite sides of the room.

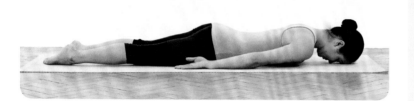

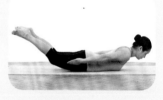

1 Lie on your front, aligning your spine and pelvis in neutral. Rest your forehead on a cushion if necessary. Lengthen your arms down by your side, palms facing up. Lengthen your legs hip-width apart, with your toes together and heels relaxed apart. Feel a gentle sense of lift in your abdominals against gravity, but make sure your shoulders and buttocks are relaxed before you begin.

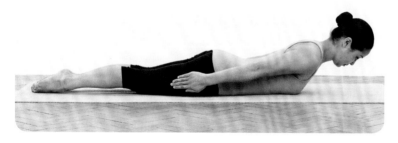

Repeat this exercise
8–10 times.

2 Breathe in to prepare and lengthen your spine. Breathe out, and begin to lift your spine, starting with the back of your head. Glide your shoulder blades into your back as your upper spine extends and your chest lifts, keeping your ribs in contact with the mat. Lift your arms and lengthen the fingertips towards your ankles, palms facing towards your body. You will feel the back of your arms activating. Simultaneously, engage your buttock and inner thighs to connect your legs and heels. Breathe in to maintain this lifted position, keeping your abdominals engaged and breathing wide into the back of the ribs. Breathe out and release back to the starting position with control. Repeat 8–10 times.

Related exercises

Dart with arm circles (pages 106–7)

Prone leg lifts

◆ GOOD FOR: Joint mobility, challenging muscles

This exercise is a great way of toning your buttock muscles and opening your hips. It also lengthens your limbs, encouraging you to work from a strong and stable centre.

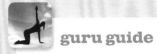

guru guide

• COMMON MISTAKES TO AVOID (see below): do not lift your leg too high nor allow your pelvis to rock to the side. Imagine your weight is even through both hip bones. The movement comes from your hip joint, not your pelvis.

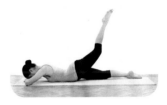

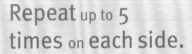

1 Lie on your front, with your spine and pelvis in neutral and feet hip-width apart with a slight turnout. Feel the front of your pelvis soft and heavy into the mat, lengthening your lower spine. Rest your forehead on your hands.

Repeat up to 5 **times** on **each side.**

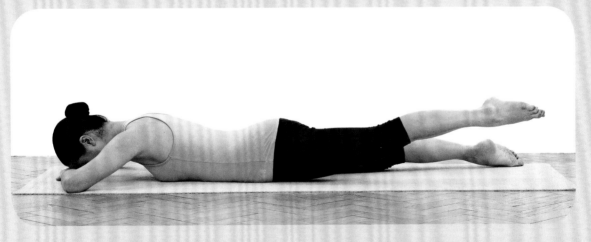

2 Breathe in to prepare and lengthen your spine. As you breathe out, deepen your abdominals and engage your buttocks to lengthen and lift one leg slightly off the mat. Think about reaching your leg back behind you rather than lifting up towards the ceiling. Keep your pelvis in neutral and your upper body relaxed and still. Breathe in to release your leg back to the mat with control. Repeat up to 5 times on each side.

Oyster

◆ GOOD FOR: Joint mobility, challenging muscles

This fantastic exercise tones your buttock muscles and challenges your core control and ability to maintain a neutral pelvis. It targets the *gluteus medius* muscle, which is a very important muscle for stabilizing your pelvis and giving your bottom a nice shape. The first variation adds challenges by working on your balance, while the second adds extra load on your buttock muscle with the extension of the leg.

For each version, repeat up to 8–10 times on each side.

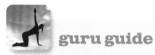

guru guide

• Do not allow your pelvis to rock back. Visualize headlights on your hip bones and make sure they continue to shine directly ahead and do not roll up to the ceiling with the movement.

• Keep your waist long and abdominals engaged throughout the movement. Imagine you are working against resistance, as if under water. Place more load on your muscles by working with precision.

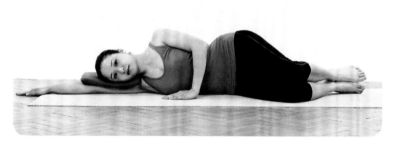

1 Lie on your side with your lower arm lengthened beneath your ear, resting your head on a pillow if necessary. Stack your shoulders, hips, knees and ankles. Find your neutral pelvis and spine. Place your top hand on the mat, palm down in front of your ribs, with your elbow bent and shoulder soft into your back. Bend your knees, and draw the feet back in line with your tailbone, feet long and toes pointing to the end of the mat.

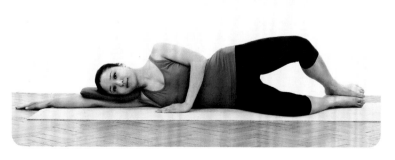

2 Breathe in to prepare and lengthen through your spine. Breathe out, deepen your connection to your centre and gently squeeze your buttock muscle to initiate the movement of your knee opening, keeping your feet together. Imagine the thighbone turning in its socket like a key in a lock. Breathe in as you lower the knee with control. Repeat up to 10 times on each side.

Oyster with foot lift

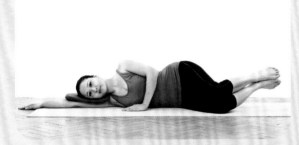

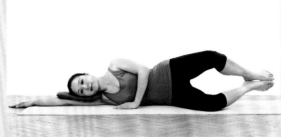

1 Start as for oyster. Breathe in to prepare and lengthen through your spine, lift both feet in line with your tailbone, keeping them together.

2 Breathe out, deepen your connection to your centre and gently squeeze your buttock muscle to start the movement of your knee opening, keeping your feet together and lifted. Breathe in to lower your knee, keeping your feet lifted. Repeat up to 8 times before changing sides.

Oyster with leg extension

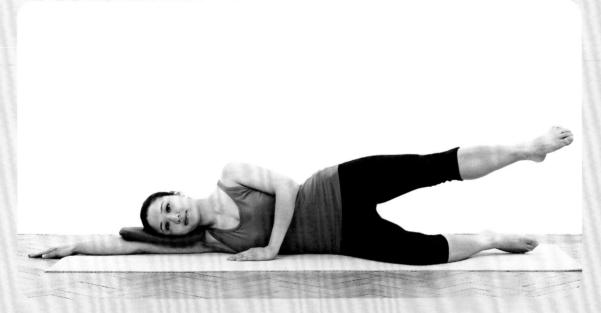

1 Start as for oyster. Breathe in to prepare and lengthen through your spine. Breathe out, deepen your connection to your centre and gently squeeze your buttock muscle to initiate opening your knee, keeping your feet together. Breathe in and extend your leg from your knee, making sure there

is no movement in the thighbone and that your knee does not dip. Keep your waist long as your toes reach away. Breathe out and bend your foot back to rest on the bottom foot. Breathe in to release your knee back down as in the starting position. Repeat up to 8 times before changing sides.

Side-lying leg kicks

◆ GOOD FOR: Joint mobility, challenging muscles

These exercises are variations of the classical side-lying exercises, adapted to build up your strength as you become familiar with the Pilates principles. They challenge your obliques and the muscles around your thighs.

Side-lying leg kicks: lift and lower

guru guide

• For the lift and lower leg kicks, try not to take your leg too high and allow your waist to dip. Keep your abdominals strong and feel your leg pressing away and out through your foot, rather than lifting too far up.

• For the front and back leg kicks, imagine you are sliding your leg along a table. Do not allow your leg to dip as it comes forward, keep the lift.

• Scoop your abdominals more as your leg travels forward, to make sure your spine does not sway with the movement.

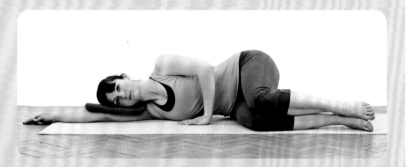

1 Lie on your side with your lower arm lengthened out underneath your ear, resting your head on a pillow if necessary. Stack your shoulders, hips, knees and ankles and find your neutral pelvis and spine. Place your top hand on the mat, palm down in front of your ribs, with your elbow bent and shoulder soft into the back. Bend your legs as if you are sitting on a chair.

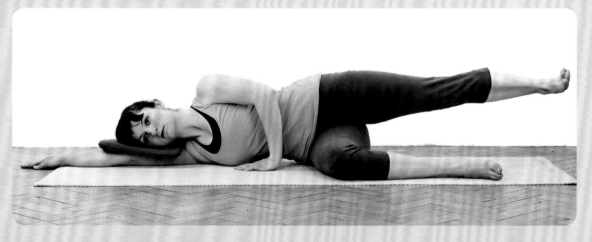

2 Breathe in to prepare and lengthen through your spine. Deepen your connection to your centre and lengthen your top leg away from your torso, in line with your hip. Flex the foot of your extended leg, pressing energy out through your heel as if you're standing on the opposite wall.

Repeat each exercise up to 10 times.

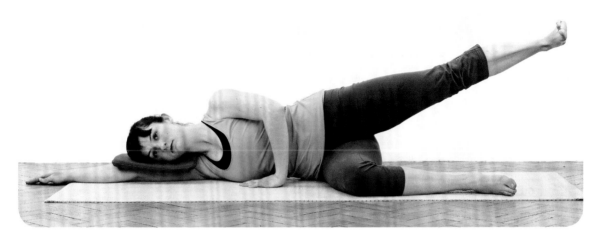

3 Breathe out as you lift your leg directly up to the ceiling, but only going as far as you are able to and still keep your waist long. Breathe in to return to the position in step 2, without resting your foot on the ground. Repeat the movement up to 10 times before changing sides.

Side-lying leg kicks: front and back

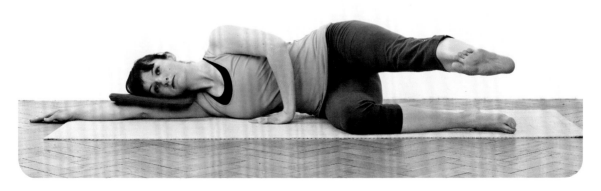

1 For step 3, breathe out as you kick the leg directly forward, only going as far as you are able to keep your spine in neutral – do not allow your bottom to swing with the movement. Breathe in to return back to the start position, without resting your foot down. Repeat up to 10 times before changing sides.

Side-lying chest openings

◆ GOOD FOR: Warming up, spinal mobility, cooling down

This is a calming exercise that mobilizes all of the spine in rotation, and encourages openness around the chest.

guru guide

• Keep your shoulder joint connected to your torso and control the opening: try not to release your arm back further than you can open your chest.

• Maintain your rib-hip connection and avoid allowing your back to arch as you twist your spine.

• Initiate the movement from your centre, not from your arm.

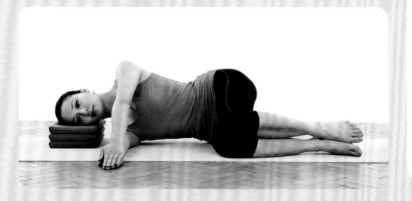

1 Lie on your side, align your spine and pelvis in neutral. Place a cushion underneath your head to bring your head and neck into line with your spine. Bend both knees in front of you as if you're sitting on a chair. Lengthen both arms on the floor, in line with your shoulders, palms together. Check that your waist is long and your centre is engaged throughout.

Repeat 8–10 times on **each side.**

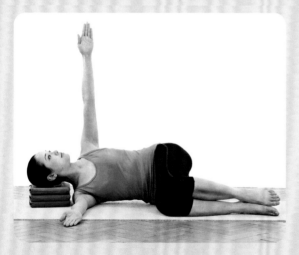

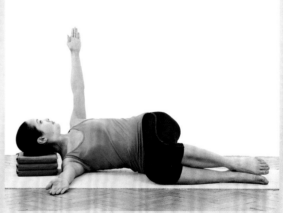

2 Breathe in to begin to float your top arm towards the ceiling, in line with your shoulder. Follow the movement of your hand with your nose as if they are connected by a magnet – begin to roll your head and turn your nose towards the ceiling as your arm lifts.

3 Breathe out to continue to open your chest and allow your arm to release back behind you, rotating from your ribcage. Make sure only your spine is moving: your hips and pelvis should stay stable. Breathe in and move your spine and arm back to centre. Breathe out to return to the start position. Repeat 8–10 times on each side.

Gluteal stretch

◆ GOOD FOR: Warming up, stretching, cooling down

This is a great way of stretching the muscles of your bottom, while challenging your neutral pelvis and spine.

Breathe into the stretch for a few breaths and repeat on the other side.

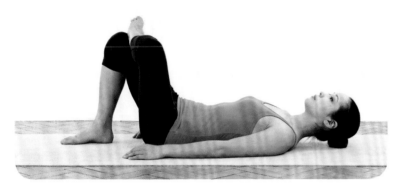

1 Lie in the relaxation position. Breathe in to prepare and lengthen your spine. Breathe out, connect to your centre and fold your left knee into your chest. Open your knee out to the side and rest your left ankle on your right knee. Breathe in, checking your neutral spine and pelvis. Check your waist is long on both sides and pelvis square.

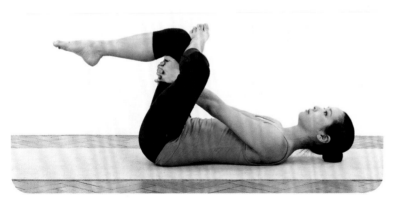

2 Breathe out, deepen your abdominals and fold your right leg in, bringing your left leg further towards you. Take your hands around the back of your right thigh, lacing your left arm between your legs. Gently draw in your right leg in and press your left knee away from you, to deepen the stretch. Make sure your tailbone stays grounded. Breathe into the stretch for a few breaths. Return your legs back down with control, and repeat on the other side.

Making it easier

Use a stretch band rather than wrapping your hands around your leg to reach it more comfortably.

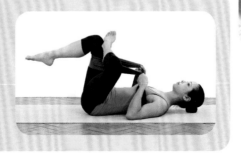

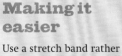 guru guide

• Make sure you do not lose neutral (page 25).

• Relax your upper body. If you feel your shoulders hunching and your neck straining, place an extra pillow underneath your head.

Pliés

◆ GOOD FOR: Warming up, joint mobility, cooling down

This ballet-inspired exercise strengthens your inner thigh and buttock muscles, mobilizes your hip, knee and ankle joints and challenges your spinal stability.

Repeat the pliés up to 10 times.

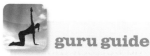

guru guide

• Gently squeeze your buttocks as you rise and make sure you don't stick your bottom out as you bend your knees. You can always hold onto a chair if this helps.

Related exercise

Pliés against a wall (page 83)

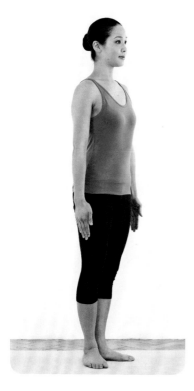

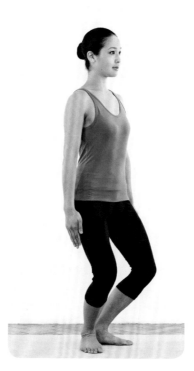

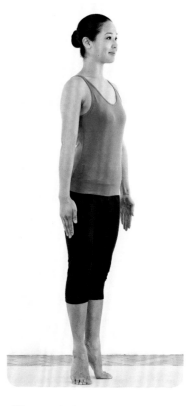

1 Stand in the Pilates stance, arms relaxed and abdominals lifted. Breathe in to prepare and lengthen through the spine.

2 Breathe out, draw your centre in and bend your knees directly over your toes. Keep your heels down to ensure most movement is from your ankle joint. Feel that the crown of your head is reaching directly up to the ceiling and that you are not tipping forward.

3 Breathe in and, maintaining a deep connection with your abdominals, draw your inner thighs together and straighten your legs. Rise onto your toes, keeping your heels together. Release your heels back down. Repeat up to 10 times.

Pliés against a wall

◆ GOOD FOR: Warming up, joint mobility, cooling down

This version of pliés offers more challenge to stability as you need to balance on one leg. It strengthens your inner thigh and buttock muscles, mobilizing your hip, knee and ankles in the correct alignment.

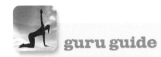

guru guide

• Feel your weight evenly through your foot and try not to allow your ankle or foot to roll inwards.

Repeat up to 8 times on each leg.

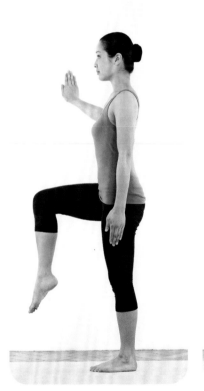

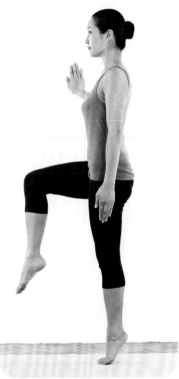

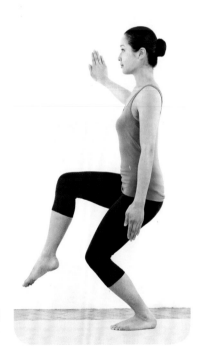

1 Stand tall, and place one hand against the wall or a chair for support. Release your weight into the leg that is furthest away from the wall. With strong abdominals, float your other leg off the floor, with your knee bent. Make sure your pelvis stays level.

2 Breathe in deeply and, as you breathe out, rise onto the toes of your supporting leg. Rise directly up with the crown of your head to the ceiling. Try not to tip your body forward as you rise. Breathe in, and slowly lower your heel back down to the floor.

3 Breathe out and bend your knee over your toes, keeping your heel on the floor. Breathe in and straighten your leg. Repeat 8 times on each leg.

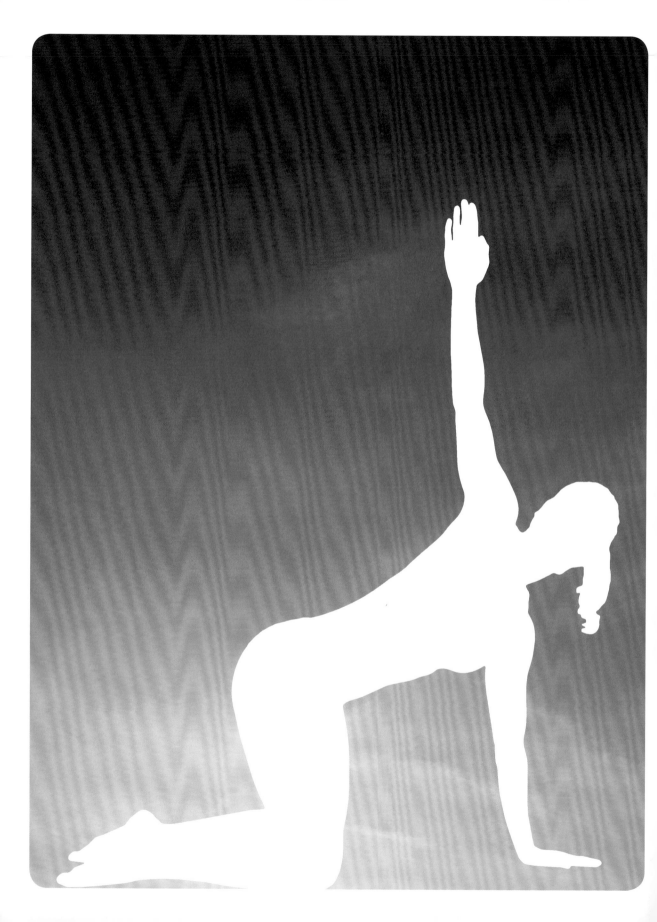

Intermediate exercises

In this section you move on to further challenge, to build on your practice so far. The level of difficulty is much greater in this section, so have patience and add challenge gradually, mixing these exercises with your basics and beginner routines while you build strength, understanding and confidence. This section begins to introduce some classical Pilates exercises, which are very challenging and bring together all Pilates principles more dynamically, to prepare you for the advanced matwork.

Mermaid

◆ GOOD FOR: Side flexion of the spine

This is a graceful exercise that lengthens your waist and challenges your oblique muscles, mobilizing your spine in side flexion with flowing movements and control. Focus on breathing into the back of your ribcage as you move.

Repeat up to 5 times on both sides.

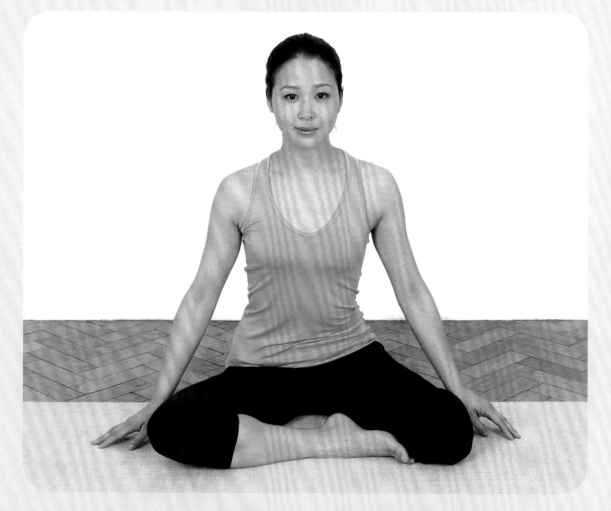

1 Sit on the mat with your left leg bent behind you and your right foot at the front touching your left knee. Make sure your knees are level and pelvis square. Soften your hands by your side and feel a sense of even heaviness through your sitting bones, even if you are slightly lifted on the left side. Lengthen evenly through both sides of the waist: try not to slump to the right. Keep your abdominals strong and shoulders level. Imagine lifting your spine up and away from your pelvis.

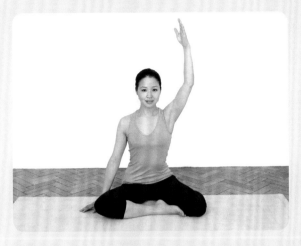

2 Breathe in to float your left arm out to the side and above your head, keeping your shoulder soft and away from your ear and your neck long.

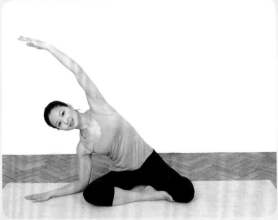

3 Breathe out and reach up and across to the right, side-bending your spine. Allow your right arm to release along the floor and bend. Keep your waist lifted on the right side. Breathe in and maintain this position, lengthening your spine and keeping your abdominals strong. You may feel a stretch along the left side of your waist. Breathe out as you lengthen your waist back to centre; allowing your right arm to straighten by your side, and floating the left arm down to rest the hand at your side.

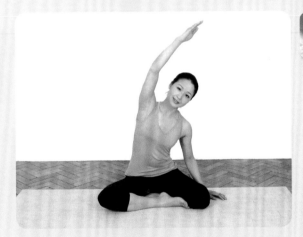

4 Breathe in to float your right arm overhead. Breathe out and lengthen up and over, bending your spine to the left. The right arm reaches in line with the spine, keeping a space between the arm and head. Keep your shoulders soft, stay long through both sides of your waist and try not to slump to the left. Breathe in and maintain your position. Breathe out to return to the centre and lower your arm to return to the start position. Repeat up to 5 times, then change the position of the legs, bringing the left leg in front, and repeat the full sequence up to 5 times on the other side.

guru guide

• COMMON MISTAKES TO AVOID (see below): try to always support the movement from your abdominals, lengthening as you side bend and keep your head in line with your spine. Try not to rotate your spine forward and collapse your chest or open your chest to arch your back. Imagine you are bending between two panes of glass.

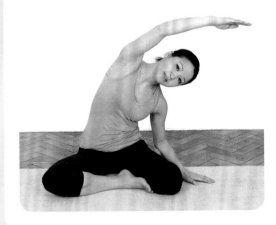

The hundred STAGE 2

◆ GOOD FOR: Challenging muscles, spinal mobility

The hundred utilizes every principle of Pilates beautifully, as seen in the preparation and stage 1 on pages 64–5. Now you learn how to challenge your deep abdominals further, coordinating with your breath and the arm beats. It takes a lot of core control, so make sure you have mastered this stage before you progress to the final stage on page 118.

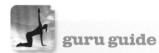

guru guide

• If you feel breathless or lightheaded, stop at once.

• Keep your neck long and relaxed throughout the exercise.

Beat your arms to a count of 100.

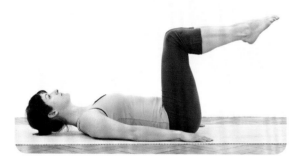

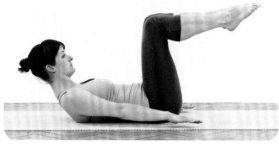

1 Lie in the relaxation position with your pelvis and spine in netural. Float one knee and then the other into a double knee fold (see page 35). Glue your feet and knees together by engaging your inner thighs.

2 Breathe in wide and full to prepare. Exhale, engage your centre and nod your chin to your chest and curl your upper body off the mat. Keep your legs still and tailbone heavy, softening your hip joints. At the same time, lengthen your arms above the floor by your sides.

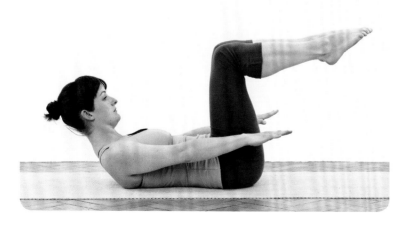

Related exercises

The hundred preparation and stages 1 and 3 (pages 64, 65 and 118)

3 Keeping your abdominals scooped, breathe in and beat your arms for a count of 5. Breathe out and again beat for a count of 5. Build up until you can repeat this 20 times (100 beats in total). Keep your eye focus down towards your navel to maintain your curl up.

Rolling like a ball

◆ GOOD FOR: Challenging muscles, spinal mobility

This fun exercise encourages smooth movement, flow and rhythm, developing your strength and control in the c-curve while massaging your spine. This is a challenging and dynamic exercise that may remind you of the freedom of movement of being a child.

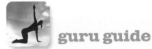

guru guide

• Imagine a magnetic connection between your nose and navel, and your heels and bottom. Maintain the space between them as you roll.

• Keep your abdominals strong to help maintain momentum.

• When tipped back in the roll, make sure you don't tip onto your neck.

Related exercises

Seal (pages 146–7)

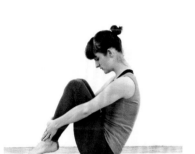

1 Sit upright on your sitting bones at one end of your mat, curl your tailbone under and deepen your abdominals to release your spine into a c-curve. Bend your knees, with your feet connected and knees slightly open. Take hold around the sides of your shins or ankles.

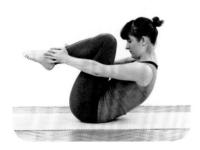

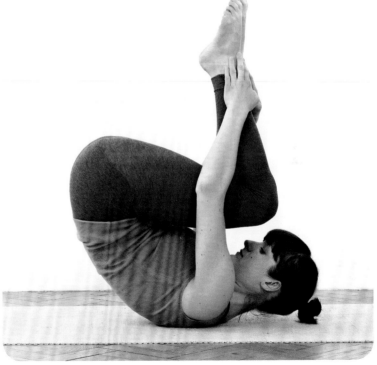

2 Tip your weight back to lift your legs slightly off the floor, and balance here. Breathe in to roll back, maintaining the c-shape of your spine and eye focus in towards your navel.

3 Once you reach the end point, around your shoulder blades, balance here momentarily if you can. Breathe out and roll back to the starting position, controlling the movement with your belly and your breath. Balance and maintain the c-curve at the top, without releasing the feet down, then roll back on the in breath. Repeat the roll up to 10 times.

Leg circles STAGE 2

◆ GOOD FOR: Joint mobility, challenging muscles

This is a progression from stage 1 on page 69. Focus on precision of movement, mobilizing your thighbone freely without allowing your torso to move. This really challenges your Pilates 'powerhouse' and uses the principles of control, precision and flowing movement.

Related exercises

Knee circles (page 68)

Leg circles: stage 1 (page 69)

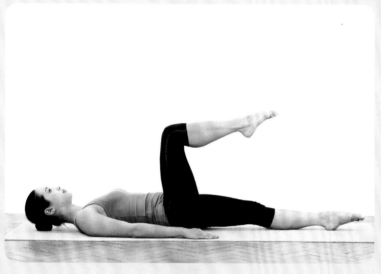

guru guide

• Make sure your pelvis and spine stays stable throughout. Feel anchored through your shoulders and ribs and let your abdominals balance your body. Your thighbone moves independently from your torso.

1 Align yourself in the relaxation position and with your spine and pelvis in neutral. Float one knee in towards your chest. Turn your leg out slightly at the hip and simultaneously lengthen the other leg away along the floor in line with your body.

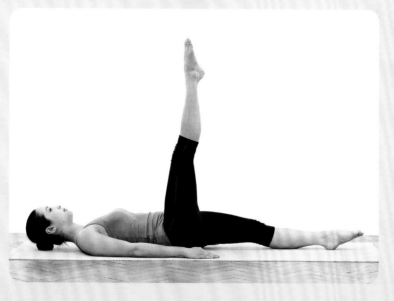

2 Lengthen your leg up towards the ceiling in its turned out position, toes softly pointed, making sure your tailbone stays heavy. Try to imagine a sense of opposition, travelling down through your thighbone into its socket, but lifted up through your toes to the ceiling.

Repeat the leg circles 5 times in each direction.

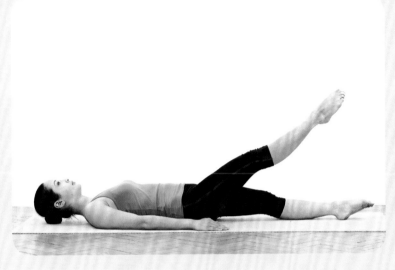

3 Deepen your abdominals to stabilize before you move. Breathe in and engage your inner thigh to draw your outstretched leg across your body, as if aiming for your opposite shoulder. Breathe out, and sweep your leg dynamically out and around, and back to the start position. Repeat 5 times in this direction, then reverse the direction.

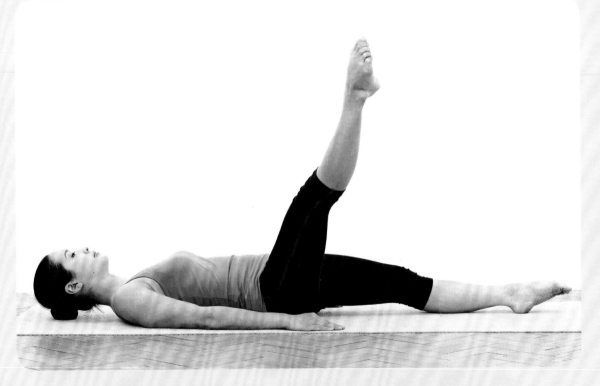

4 Breathe in to release your leg away from your body, taking it as wide as your shoulder and no further. Breathe out, lower your leg across your body and sweep it around and up, back to the starting position. Repeat 5 times in this direction. Lower your leg to the mat, and repeat on the other leg.

Single leg stretch STAGE 2

◆ GOOD FOR: Challenging muscles, spinal and joint mobility, stretching

This is the progression from stage 1 (see page 66), with added challenge for your abdominals. You will need to be able to coordinate your breath with the smooth, flowing movement of your limbs from a strong centre.

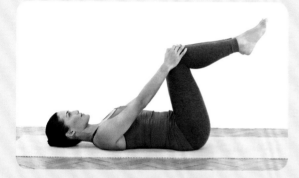

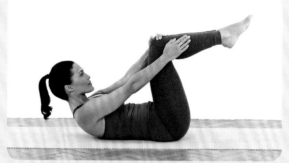

1 Lie in the relaxation position, with your pelvis and spine in neutral. Breathe in wide and full to prepare. As you breathe out, gently engage your centre and double knee fold your legs towards your chest (see page 35).

2 Breathe in, and take your left hand across your right knee. Extend your right hand down the side of your shin. Keep your elbows open and shoulders relaxed. Breathe out, deepen your abdominals and curl your head and shoulders off the mat, directing your eye focus toward your navel.

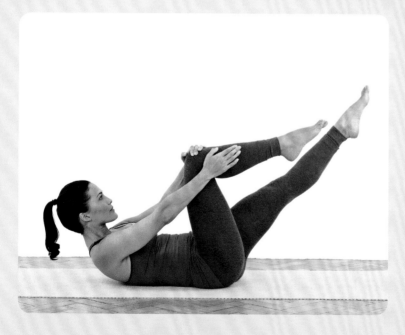

> *Related exercises*
>
> Single leg stretch: stages 1 and 3 (pages 66 and 119)

3 Breathe out, deepen your abdominals and straighten your left leg, at about a 45-degree angle. Make sure your leg isn't too low, keep your back anchored to the floor and maintain the neutral position of your pelvis.

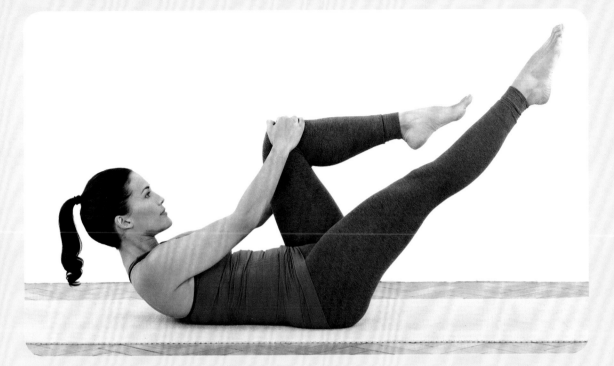

4 Breathe in and bend your knee back in, then change your hand position onto your left knee. Breathe out and extend the right leg. Repeat up to 10 times on each leg.

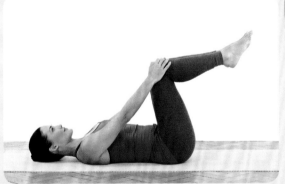

5 On an out breath, curl your head and shoulders back down to the floor with control, then float your legs individually back down. Once this stage becomes easy, you are ready to progress to stage 3, on page 119.

Repeat up to **10 times** on **each leg.**

 guru guide

• Keep your eye focus central, and avoid 'bobbing' your head from side to side as you move your legs.

• Keep your torso still and strong.

• COMMON MISTAKES TO AVOID (see below): make sure you lengthen your leg with control, try not to allow it to fall too far to the floor and hang from your spine.

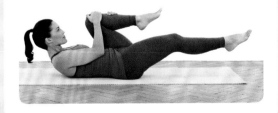

Spine stretch forward

◆ GOOD FOR: Challenging muscles, stretching, spinal mobility

This exercise strengthens the c-curve and mobilizes your spine with a long, lifted waist, challenging your deep abdominals as you move slowly and with control. It also develops an awareness of deep lateral breathing.

Related exercises

C-curve (page 39)

Saw (pages 114–15)

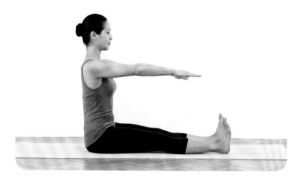

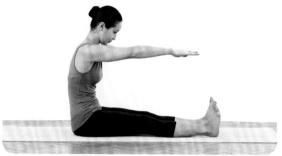

1 Sit upright with your legs straight out in front of you, about shoulder-width apart and in parallel with your kneecaps facing the ceiling. Flex your feet. Find your neutral pelvis and spine and activate the deep abdominals. Release your arms ahead of you in line with your shoulders or slightly lower, palms facing down.

2 Breathe into your ribcage and lengthen your spine. Breathe out and lengthen your spine forward, rolling bone by bone. Curl forward by imagining someone pulling you from your fingertips as you resist and draw back with your abdominals. Keep your legs active and pressing forward through your heels.

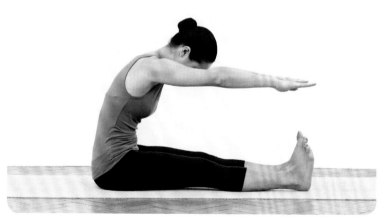

guru guide

• Make sure you don't roll your pelvis forward. You should be able to feel the sitting bones heavy into the mat throughout.

• Use your breath to try to go deeper into the stretch.

• Keep your shoulders softly connected to your body, try not to hunch your shoulders.

3 Roll forward slowly, with your eye focus to your knees and the crown of your head releasing forward as you curl your spine. Keep your arms level with your ears and your neck long. Breathe in and begin to restack your spine to neutral, initiating the movement from your centre. Repeat up to 5 times.

Spine twist

◆ GOOD FOR: Challenging muscles, spinal mobility

This is a classical exercise, focusing on great abdominal control as you twist your spine with length and stability.

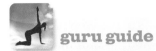

guru guide

• Make sure your pelvis does not move: one foot should not move forward as you twist, they should remain level with your sitting bones even on the floor.

• Deepen your abdominals as you twist, turning from your waist not your arms.

• Avoid arching your back or leaning backwards as you twist. You should twist around a straight line, as if around a pole.

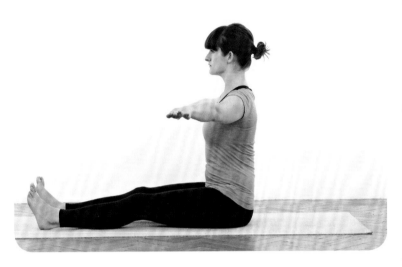

1 Sit up tall with your legs outstretched in front of you, feet flexed and your legs connected and in parallel. Find your neutral pelvis and spine, and make sure you are even on your sitting bones. Raise your arms to the sides, within your peripheral vision, palms facing down and fingers lengthened. Breathe in to prepare and lengthen the spine.

Repeat up to 5 times in each direction.

Related exercise
Saw (pages 114–15)

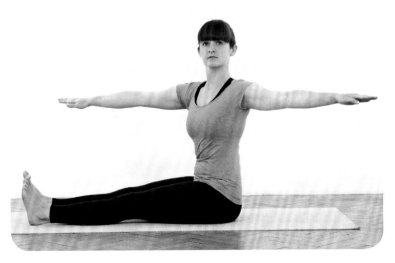

2 Breathe out and turn your head to the left, deepen your abdominals and begin to twist your torso, imagining you are spiralling upwards with the crown of your head and lifting your ribcage from your pelvis. Allow your eye focus to travel over your shoulder to complete the twist of your neck. End with a double pulse into the full rotation, to expel the air from your lungs. Breathe in to return your spine to the start. Repeat to the other side. Repeat up to 5 times in each direction.

Scissors

◆ GOOD FOR: Challenging muscles, stretching, spinal and joint mobility

Part of the classical mat, this is a tough exercise. You will strengthen your abdominals and legs and stretch your hamstrings dynamically, while working on your coordination and control. Have fun working with the swift movement.

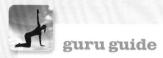

guru guide

• Make sure you do not lose neutral when lowering and raising your legs.

• Relax your upper body. Do not pull your leg in with your arms, allow your hands just to guide your leg. Make sure your belly does the work.

• Do not allow your back to rock on the mat, keep strong and anchored through your ribcage and tailbone.

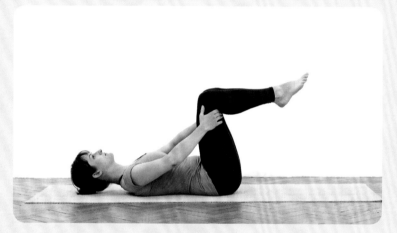

1 Lie in the relaxation position. On an out breath, fold both knees into your chest. Take hold of your right leg behind your thigh, with elbows wide and chest open. Breathe in to prepare and lengthen your spine.

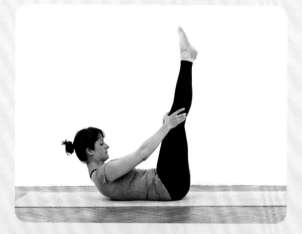

2 Breathe out, connect to your centre and straighten both legs towards the ceiling, toes softly pointed. Take your hands as far up your right leg as you can reach without hunching your shoulders. Keep your elbows soft and open. Breathe in as you deepen your belly and curl your head and shoulders off the mat.

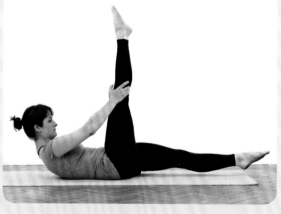

3 Breathe out and scoop your belly more as you lengthen your left leg down towards the floor, stopping before you reach the floor. Have your leg long and straight and toes softly pointed. Feel your hamstring muscles working as you lower the leg, and avoid gripping the front of your thigh.

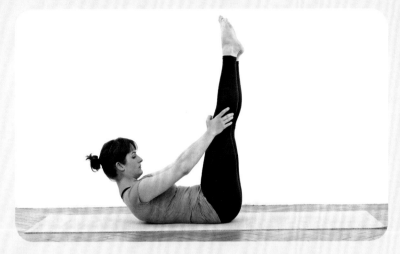

Related exercise

Climb a tree (pages 136–7)

Repeat up to 8 times on each leg.

4 Breathe in to raise your leg, keeping it as straight as you can, lifting it with your abdominals. Make sure your pelvis stays in neutral throughout.

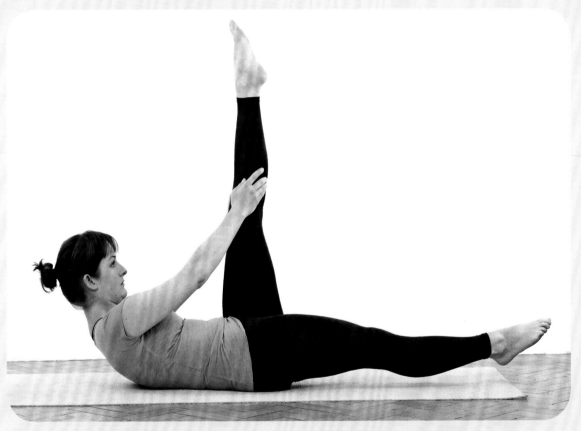

5 Breathe out and change your hand position to your left leg, and lower the right leg with control. Keep your abdominals strong and your shoulders soft throughout. Keep your eye focus towards your centre. Repeat up to 8 times on each leg. To finish the exercise, fold both knees back into your chest and release your head and shoulders to the floor with control. Return to the relaxation position on an out breath.

Coordination

◆ GOOD FOR: Challenging muscles, spinal and joint mobility

This is one of Pilates' apparatus exercises, adapted to make a challenging and dynamic matwork exercise. Instead of springs for your muscles to work against, you need to create the resistance for your muscles with your control of the movement.

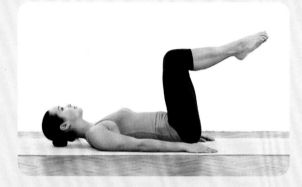

1 Lie in the relaxation position and double knee fold your legs in towards your chest using your abdominals, toes together and knees apart.

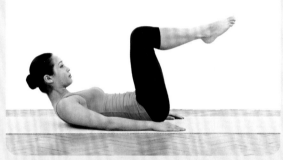

2 On an out breath, deepen your belly and curl your head and shoulders off the mat, your forehead releasing towards your knees.

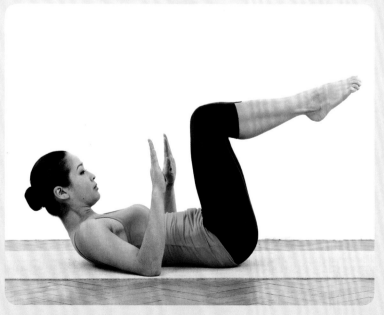

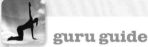

guru guide

• Do not allow your back to arch. Keep your abdominals scooped throughout and feel anchored into the mat.

Repeat up to 5 times.

3 Bend your elbows and raise your forearms so your palms face forward, vertical to the floor.

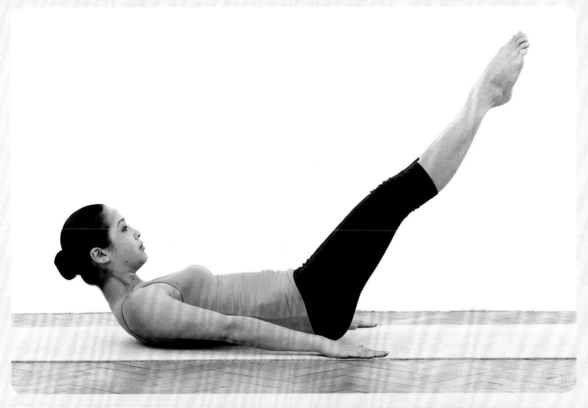

4 Breathe in and connect deeply to your centre as you press your legs away from your body in the Pilates stance. Lengthen your arms forward and place your palms on the floor. Take your legs only as low as you can control them with your abdominals and avoid your back arching.

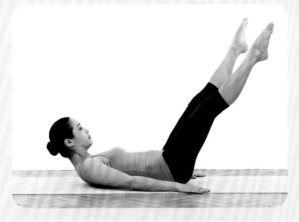

5 Breathe out and swiftly open and close your legs, using your inner thighs. Take them only as wide as your shoulders. Imagine your legs are glued together and you must strongly pull them apart. Deepen the engagement of your abdominals as you beat your legs.

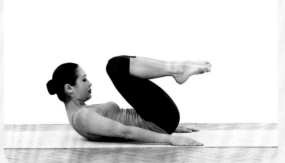

6 Breathe in and bend your knees towards your chest, using your belly to draw them deeply towards you. Curl up further as your legs come in. Breathe out and bend your elbows to bring your arms back to the starting position. Repeat up to 5 times.

Spine curls: progression

◆ GOOD FOR: Challenging muscles, spinal and joint mobility

Adding challenge to the spine curls on page 34, these curls mobilize your spine and strengthen your back, buttocks and legs, requiring greater coordination and balance.

Related exercise

Spine curls (page 34)

Spine curls with arms

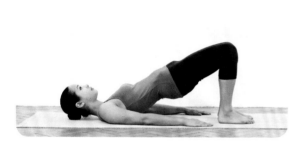

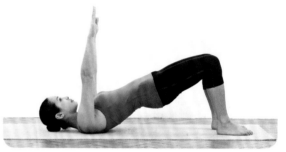

1 Align yourself in the relaxation position. Breathe in wide into your back and lengthen your spine. Breathe out and curl your tailbone under, rolling your lower spine into the mat and continuing to peel bone by bone until you reach your shoulder blades.

2 Breathe in and maintain this position with strength, as you float your arms up above your shoulders.

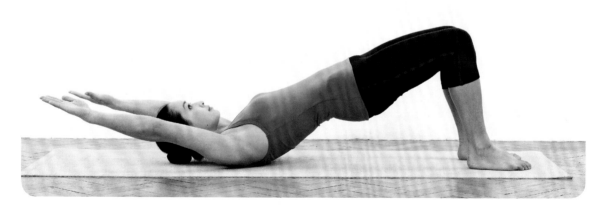

3 Release your arms back behind your head. Keep them in line with your ears and try not to force them down to the ground. Maintain a strong abdominal connection between your ribcage and hips to avoid arching your back – think of your ribcage closure (see page 30). Breathe out and, leaving your arms behind you, wheel your spine back down to the mat, softening equally through every section of your spine. When your tailbone reaches the mat, breathe in and float your arms up and release them back down by your sides. Repeat up to 10 times.

Spine curls with leg extension

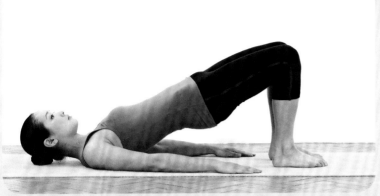

guru guide

• Be very careful not to allow your pelvis to dip from one side to the other as you extend your leg.

• As your arms come up, do not allow your hips to dip. Stay in a strong line from your shoulders out to your knees.

1 Align yourself in the relaxation position. Breathe in wide into your back and lengthen your spine. Breathe out and curl your tailbone under, rolling your lower spine into the mat and continuing to peel bone by bone until you reach your shoulder blades.

Repeat up to 5 times.

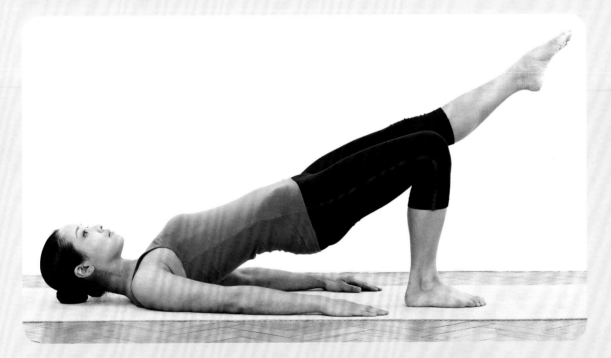

2 Breathe in and maintain this position with strength. Stand strong into one foot as you extend your opposite leg, keeping your knees level with each other. Make sure your hips do not dip – engage your centre and buttocks strongly to ensure your torso stays lifted.

Breathe in and release your foot down. Breathe out, and extend the other leg. Stay relaxed and heavy across your shoulders and arms. Float the foot down on your in breath, and as you breathe out release your spine down to the mat, bone by bone. Repeat up to 5 times.

The half teaser

◆ GOOD FOR: Challenging muscles, spinal and joint mobility

This exercise builds strength for the teaser (see pages 138–9), developing the control and stability needed for the advanced exercise. The half teaser requires great abdominal strength and balance.

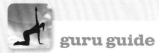

guru guide

• Make sure that your chest doesn't slump forward: feel you are opening your chest and showing your breastbone towards your toes.

• Try not to reach your arms too far, keep your neck long and shoulders connected softly to your body.

• Keep your legs strong and active throughout the exercise.

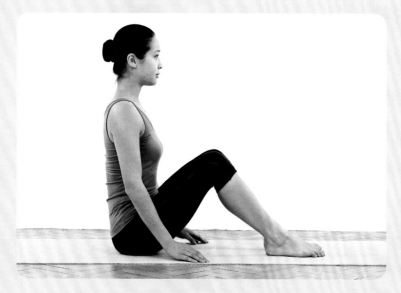

1 Sit up tall with your legs together, feet flat on the floor. Find your neutral pelvis and spine and gently engage your abdominals before you begin.

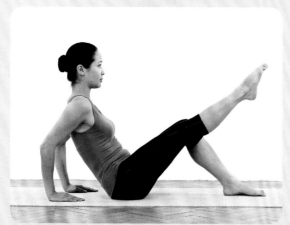

2 Breathe in, deepen your abdominal connection and curl your spine back slightly, using your arms for support. Breathe out and lengthen one leg from your hip, keeping your knees connected.

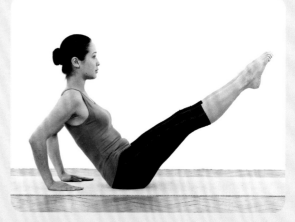

3 Breathe in, extend your second leg and find your balance, turning up the engagement of your centre to hold the weight of your legs.

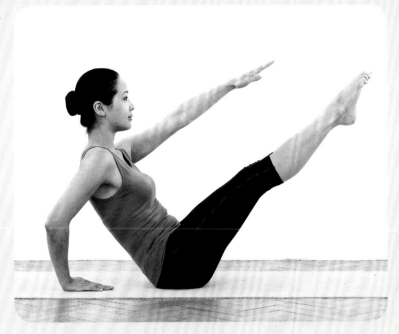

Related exercise

The teaser (pages 138–9)

Repeat up to 8 times.

4 Breathe out to release one arm forward, fingertips reaching towards your toes. Make sure you haven't allowed your chest to slump and your spine to change shape. Keep your chest open and abdominals working, and your legs strong by connecting your inner thighs. Try not to allow your legs to dip.

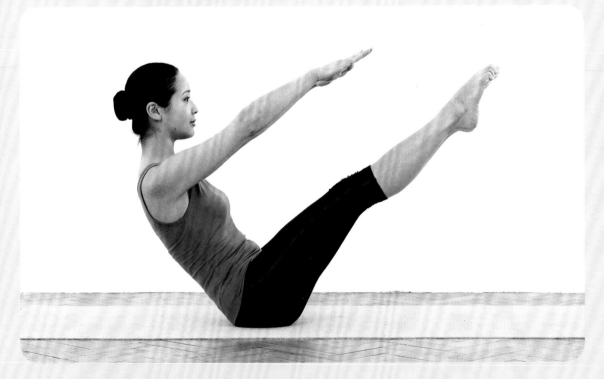

5 On the same out breath, reach your second arm forward so you are in a letter 'V' with your body and your arms are parallel with your legs. Breathe in to release your arms slowly back to the mat, then bend one leg followed by the other. Repeat up to 8 times, then roll back into your relaxation position.

Cobra

◆ GOOD FOR: Challenging muscles, spinal mobility

This classical exercise is inspired by yoga, and mobilizes the spine sequentially in extension, strengthening your back, toning your abdominals and opening your hips.

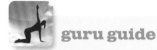

guru guide

• Don't collapse into your lower back – keep your abdominals lifted and centre strong and feel length throughout.

• Keep your neck long, shoulders soft away from your ears and don't compress your spine.

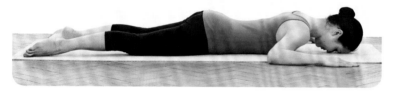

1 Align yourself on your front with your spine and pelvis in neutral. Rest your forehead on the mat and have your arms bent wide by your sides, palms down, thumbs in line with your nose. Allow your shoulders to relax and feel open across your chest. Gently engage your abdominals before you begin.

Related exercises

Cobra preparation (page 37)

Swan dive (pages 128–9)

Swimming (page 130)

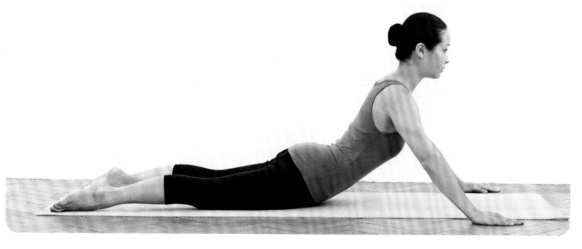

2 Breathe in and peel the spine off the mat as on page 37. Release your forehead up, then your breastbone, ribcage and abdominals. Roll all the way up to the front of your pelvis, feeling your hip joints opening and strongly engage your abdominals. Breathe out and begin to lower your spine sequentially in reverse. Repeat up to 8 times. When you have finished the exercise, press yourself back into the rest position to release your spine in the opposite direction.

Double leg lifts

◆ GOOD FOR: Challenging muscles, joint mobility

This exercise opens the front of your hips, working the buttocks and challenging the stability of your pelvis and spine. This and the cobra are the preparation exercises to develop strength for the swan dive on pages 128–9.

Related exercises

Prone leg lifts (page 75)

Swan dive (pages 128–9)

Swimming (page 130)

Repeat up to **10** times.

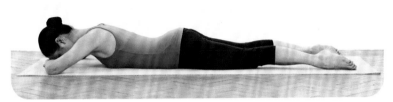

1 Align yourself on your front and rest your forehead on your hands. Relax your shoulders, keep your collarbones wide and find your neutral pelvis and spine. Lengthen your legs away, hip-width apart and turned out. Gently engage your centre before you begin. Breathe in to prepare and lengthen through your spine.

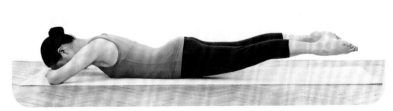

2 Breathe out, lengthen and then lift both legs slightly off the mat. Think about reaching your legs away behind you rather than lifting them high. Feel your hips lengthening and opening across the front with an even weight on your hip bones. Allow your shoulders to stay soft. Breathe in to lengthen your legs back to the floor. Repeat up to 10 times.

guru guide

• Always keep your abdominals lifted to support your lower back.

• Keep the turnout from your hip joint as you reach your legs, do not allow them to relax into parallel.

• COMMON MISTAKES TO AVOID (see right): try not to allow your knees to bend. Keep your legs straight and buttocks working.

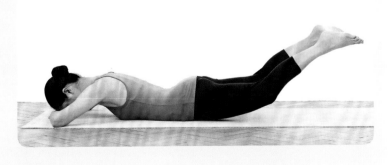

Dart with arm circles

◆ GOOD FOR: Challenging muscles, spinal and joint mobility

This exercise strengthens your spine and tones your legs and buttocks, coordinating flowing movement with timing of the arm circles. This is a progression from the dart (see page 74), adding challenge with extra load on your upper back muscles from circling your arms.

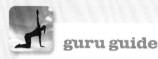

guru guide

• Keep your feet on the floor throughout the exercise and keep your pelvis stable.

• Make sure you keep your eye focus down: do not allow the back of your neck to shorten and look forward.

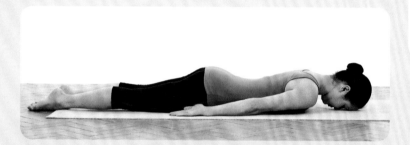

1 Align yourself on the mat on your front, with your spine and pelvis in neutral. Rest your forehead on a pillow on the mat. Have your arms by your sides, palms facing up, and shoulders relaxed so that you feel open across your chest. Your legs are in parallel and inner thighs connected, toes pointed. Gently connect to your centre.

Related exercise

Dart (page 74)

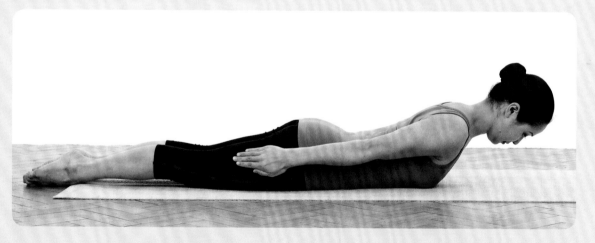

2 Breathe in wide and full to prepare and lengthen your spine. Breathe out, lift your abdominals and begin to lengthen the crown of your head forward. Open your collarbones and glide your shoulder blades into your back to lift your upper spine from the mat. Simultaneously lengthen your arms, rotating them so your palms face your thighs. Imagine you are reaching your fingers to your ankles. Keep your eye focus down to the mat and lengthen your toes along the floor.

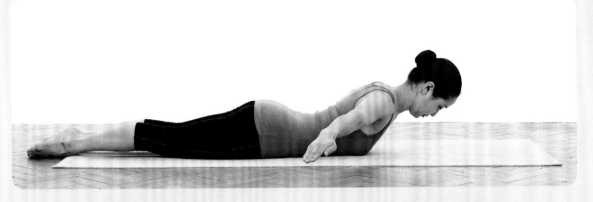

3 Breathe in, stay lifted through your upper back and keep your abdominals strong as you begin to open your arms out by your sides, as if you were a bird spreading your wings. Make sure you move both arms at the same time, keep them at shoulder level and turn your palms to face the floor.

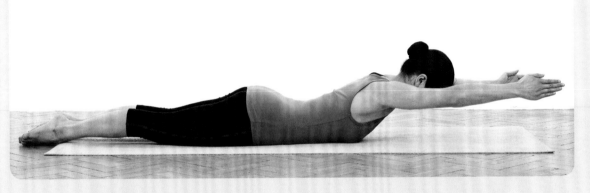

4 Continue to circle your arms up and above your head, shoulder-width apart, palms facing towards each other. Focus on lengthening your body from head to toe, rather than lifting too high and arching your back.

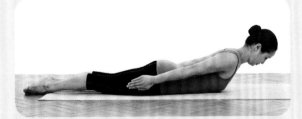

5 Breathe out and reverse the circle, taking your arms back down by your sides. Feel your spine extending slightly further as you reach back. Maintain your eye focus towards the mat and a soft tuck of the chin to your chest.

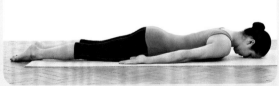

6 Breathe in and slowly return your body back to the mat. Repeat up to 8 times. Press yourself back into your rest position to release the spine in the opposite direction from that you have just worked in.

Torpedo

◆ GOOD FOR: Challenging muscles, joint mobility

This exercise works your waist muscles and demands good balance. A lot of core strength is required to lift the weight of your legs off the floor without rocking your torso. There are two stages. Practise the first before progressing.

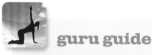

guru guide

• When you are aligning your body for step 1, hinge from the hips and bring them slightly in front if you need some help with your balance.

• Make sure your legs are either in line with your body or slightly forward. They should not be reaching behind you.

• Keep your waist lengthened and lifted so there is a lightness or space underneath your waist. Keep those obliques working.

• Feel your body lengthening out from the crown of your head through to your toes.

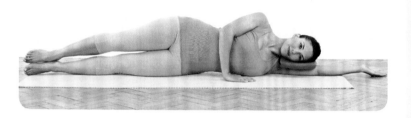

1 Align yourself on your side, with your legs straight and lengthened in line with your body and your toes softly pointed. Lengthen your left arm under your head in line with your body. Bend your top arm in front of you to give you some support – but do not rest all your weight on your hand. Keep your chest open and shoulder blade soft into your back.

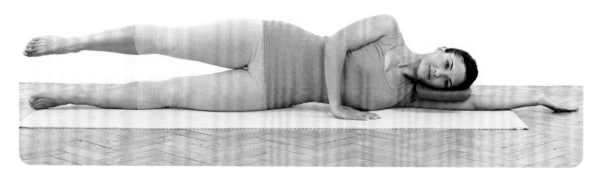

2 Breathe in to prepare and lengthen your spine. Breathe out, connect to your centre and raise your top leg. Think about reaching it away from you rather than lifting it to the ceiling. Keep your waist long and pelvis stable.

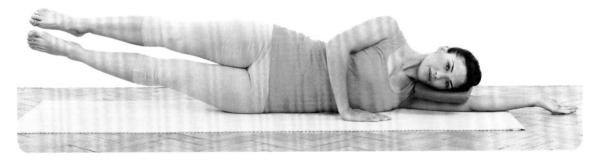

3 Breathe in and, keeping your abdominals strong, lift your lower leg to join the top one, feeling your waist, inner thighs and buttocks working. Do not allow your back to arch or waist to collapse onto the mat.

Repeat up to 10 times on each side.

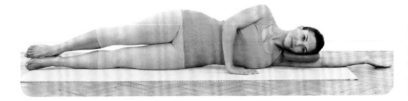

4 Breathe out and slowly lower both legs back down to the floor together. Resist the movement with your lower leg, to encourage your muscles to work. Repeat up to 10 times on each side.

Making it harder

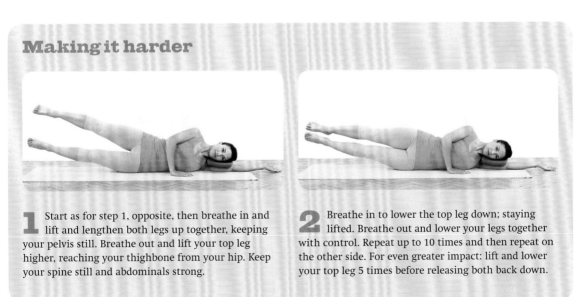

1 Start as for step 1, opposite, then breathe in and lift and lengthen both legs up together, keeping your pelvis still. Breathe out and lift your top leg higher, reaching your thighbone from your hip. Keep your spine still and abdominals strong.

2 Breathe in to lower the top leg down; staying lifted. Breathe out and lower your legs together with control. Repeat up to 10 times and then repeat on the other side. For even greater impact: lift and lower your top leg 5 times before releasing both back down.

Thread the needle

◆ GOOD FOR: Challenging muscles, stretching, spinal mobility

This exercise mobilizes your spine in rotation, challenging your control and balance. It also strengthens the deep stabilizing muscles of the shoulder area and stretches your upper back. Thread the needle with arm openings adds further challenge, requiring more balance and stability. It is also a lovely way of opening your chest. With both versions of thread the needle, keep the movement flowing.

guru guide

• Keep your abdominals strong throughout the rotation.

• Focus on keeping your spine long and your waist long on either side, trying not to dip your hips, arch your back or curl your tailbone under. Allow the rotation to come from your ribcage not from your hips.

• Maintain space between your shoulders and ears throughout.

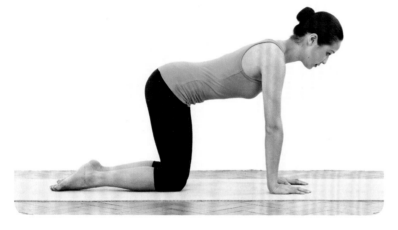

1 Align yourself on your mat in four-point kneeling, pelvis and spine in neutral. Engage your deep abdominal muscles and connect your shoulders into your body. Keep your neck long.

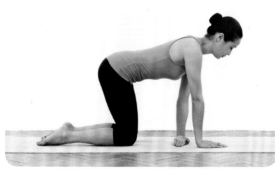

2 Breathe in to prepare and lengthen your spine. Transfer your weight onto your right hand. Breathe out, engage your centre and lift your left hand, placing the back of your hand onto the mat.

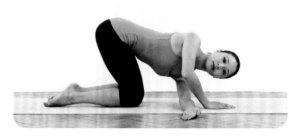

3 Slide the back of your hand along the mat, under your right arm, in line with your breastbone, allowing your spine to twist sequentially. Bend your right arm to allow the ribcage to move. Let your head follow the movement of your spine, turning to face your right hand. Breathe in to return to centre. Either alternate sides, or repeat on the same side, 8 times on each.

Thread the needle with arm openings

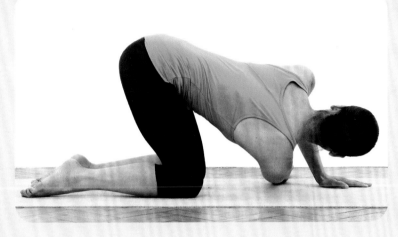

1 Follow steps 1–3 for thread the needle. When you return to your starting position with your in breath, continue to bring your arm out to the side of your body.

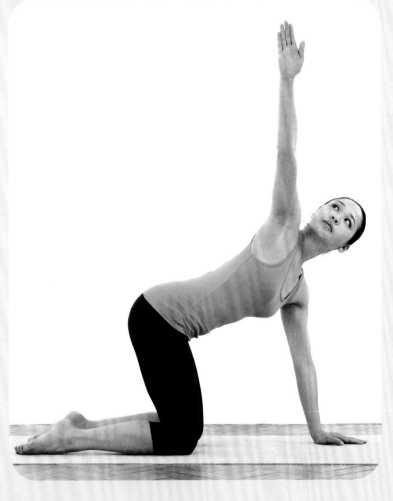

Repeat up to
8 times on **each side.**

2 Breathe out to open your arm up to the ceiling, twisting your spine to follow the movement and rotating your head to the right. Open across your chest and shoulders. Release your fingers to the ceiling, but only open your arm as far as you can open your chest. Repeat up to 8 times on each side.

Cat to down dog

◆ GOOD FOR: Challenging muscles, stretching, spinal and joint mobility

This flowing sequence strengthens your arms and stretches your spine and the backs of your legs, encouraging you to coordinate your abdominals with spinal movement. It is an energizing exercise, fluidly combining Pilates with a yoga influence.

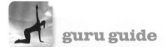

guru guide

• Keep your neck long and maintain the space between your shoulders and ears: try not to hunch your shoulders, keep them drawn into your back.

• Keep your weight even on both hands and feet.

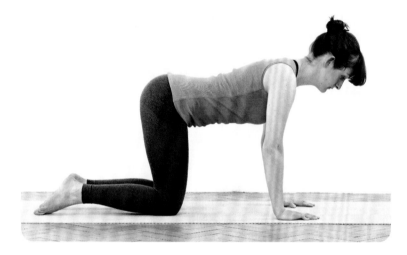

Repeat up to 10 times.

1 Align yourself on the mat in four-point kneeling, spine in neutral and abdominals gently engaged.

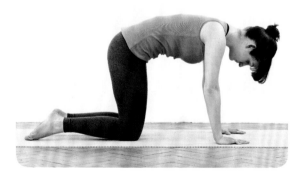

2 Breathe in to prepare and lengthen through your spine. Breathe out, and curl your tailbone under to sequentially roll your spine into a c-curve cat position.

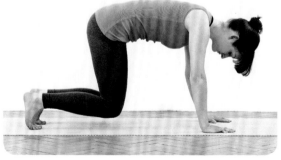

3 On the same out breath, if possible, lift your knees off the mat and begin to straighten your legs, maintaining the c-shape of the spine for as long as possible.

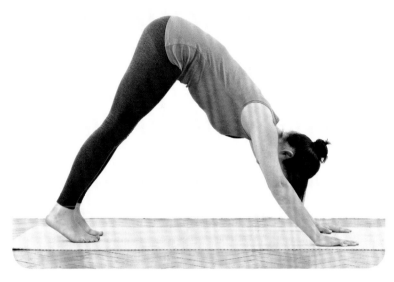

4 Breathe in as you feel the stretch in the back of your legs and actively lengthen your spine, reaching your tailbone up towards the ceiling. Press strongly into your hands, opening your shoulder joints and releasing your heels down. Draw your abdominals deeply in towards your spine. Allow your eye focus to naturally release to the floor below your navel.

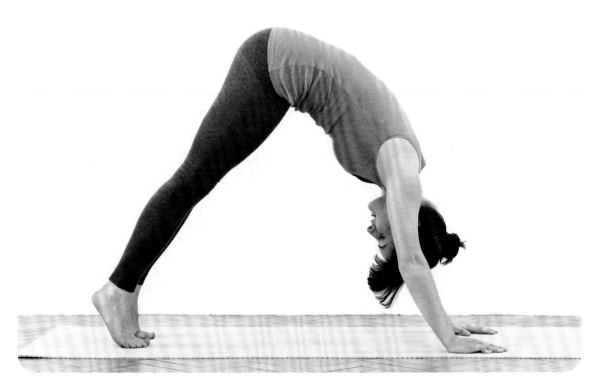

5 Breathe out and rise onto the balls of your feet, beginning to flex the spine once more into your c-curve. Continue to breathe out as you bring your knees back down to the floor beneath your hips, back into the cat position of the spine, abdominals lifted. Breathe in and lengthen your spine back to neutral. Repeat up to 10 times.

Saw

◆ GOOD FOR: Challenging muscles, stretching, spinal mobility

This movement really encourages the Pilates breath, developing an effective technique by encouraging you to 'wring out the lungs' with the rotation and forward bend to get the most out of the movement. It also stretches your spine and back of your legs, and challenges pelvic stability.

Repeat to each side up to 5 times.

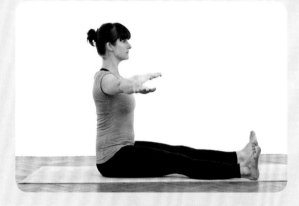 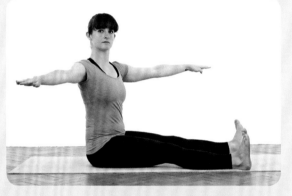

1 Sit up tall on the mat, pelvis and spine in neutral and weight even on both sitting bones. Open your feet just wider than the width of the mat and with your kneecaps facing up to the ceiling and feet flexed. Lengthen your arms out to the side, at shoulder height, palms facing down, fingers long. Draw in your abdominals to strengthen the spine and feel your ribcage lift away from your pelvis.

2 Breathe in and twist your body to the right, rotating fully from your navel up to your nose. Allow your arms to twist as far as your body, keeping them in line with your shoulders. Look towards your middle finger.

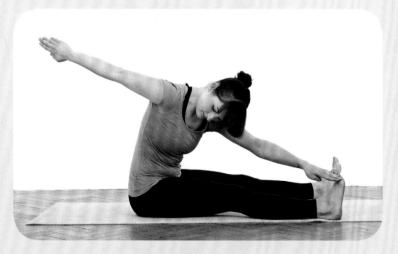

3 Breathe out and nod your chin to your chest. Curl forward over your right leg, ensuring your spine is twisting. Reach your left arm across your right leg as if you are trying to saw off your little toe, palm facing down. At the same time, open your right shoulder to reach your right arm behind you, pressing your palm away in the opposite direction to increase the twist, reaching with your fingertips. Look towards your right hip as you pulse your left arm forward 3 times over or beyond your foot to increase the twist of your spine, expelling all the air from your lungs with each pulse.

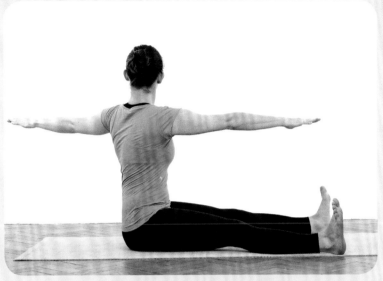

guru guide

• Make sure your pelvis does not move: check whether your feet are shifting position as you twist. If they are, deepen your centre connection and lift your movement from your ribcage, keeping your pelvis heavy and grounded, pressing out through your heels and keeping the sitting bones still.

• When you are pulsing in step 3, do not collapse your upper body – keep your abdominals lifted and strong. Coordinate the breath with the movement.

4 Breathe in to roll up through your spine and twist back to the centre. Then twist across to the left.

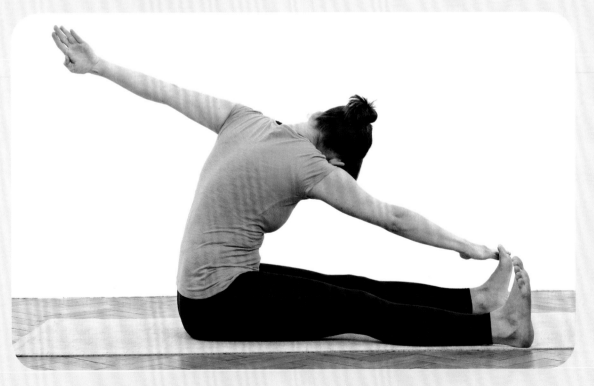

5 Breathe out as you curl forward over the left leg, reaching your right arm across to saw off your little toe, reaching with your arms and pulsing forward three times. Breathe in to restack. Repeat to each side up to 5 times and then return to the starting position and relax your arms down by your sides.

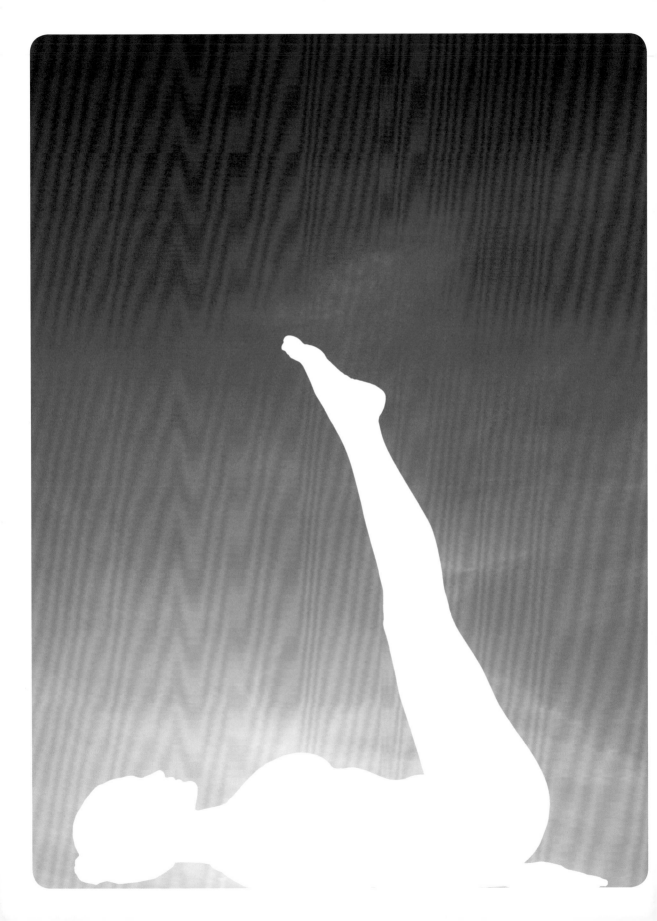

Advanced exercises

Here are some of the ultimate challenges within the Pilates matwork repertoire. Once you have mastered the intermediate exercises and feel strong and confident in your practice, you are ready to move on and take on more of the classical work. Some of the exercises described here take years of practise to master. They continue to evolve and often challenge your understanding of Pilates as a technique, so be patient and see this as the beginning of your Pilates journey.

The hundred STAGE 3

◆ GOOD FOR: Challenging muscles, spinal and joint mobility

This exercise challenges the abdominals and leg muscles, builds stamina and encourages freedom of movement around your shoulders. Deep lateral breathing and the pumping arm movement warms up your body.

guru guide

• Keep your eye focus down and into your navel. Ensure your neck is long and head still, trying not to bounce through your torso and staying soft in your neck and shoulders.

Related exercises

The hundred: stages 1 and 2 (pages 64–5 and 88–9)

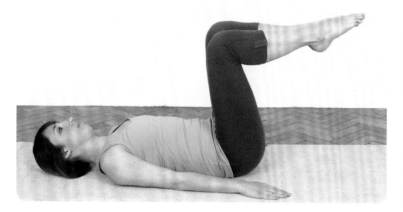

1 Lie in the relaxation position. Float both knees into your chest, one by one. Keep your heels connected, toes softly pointed and knees shoulder-width apart. Breathe in to prepare and lengthen your spine.

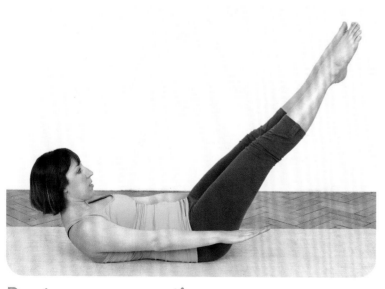

2 As you breathe out, nod your chin to your chest, engage your pelvic floor and abdominals and curl into the curl-up position. Lengthen your arms forward, reaching right through your fingers. At the same time, straighten your legs to around a 45-degree angle, thighs connected in Pilates stance. Deepen the abdominal connection. Breathe in for a count of 5 and beat your arms. Repeat, breathing out for a count of 5. Do this 10 times up to a count of 100. To finish, stay curled up, bend your knees into your chest. Keep your abdominals strong and lower your feet one by one, returning to the relaxation position.

Beat your arms 100 times.

Single leg stretch STAGE 3

◆ GOOD FOR: Challenging muscles, stretching, spinal and joint mobility

The advanced stage of this dynamic exercise moves more swiftly with the breath pattern than stage 2 (see pages 92–3), developing your stamina and coordination. It is one of the most effective abdominal exercises there is!

> *Related exercises*
>
> Single leg stretch: stages 1 and 2 (pages 66 and 92–3)

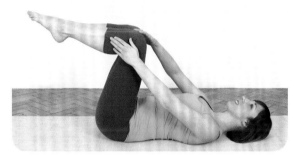 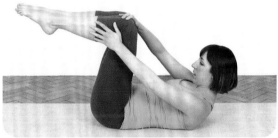

1 Lie in the relaxation position. Float both knees into your chest. Place your right hand around your left knee, and your left hand down the side of your shin. Legs are hip-width apart.

2 As you breathe out, nod your chin to your chest and curl into the curl-up position. Keep your abdominals strong and pelvis grounded and in neutral the whole time you are in this position.

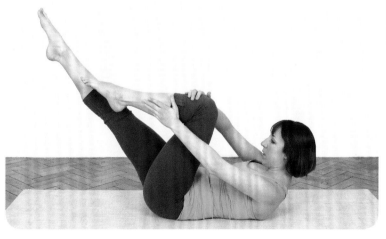

 guru guide

• Keep your neck long: make sure your head is still and your eye focus is towards the abdominals and central through the legs – do not bend your head from side to side with the leg change.

• Keep your arms strong, draw your knees in towards your chest using your arm muscles actively. Allow the movements to be smooth and flowing.

3 Breathe in deeply, then breathe out and draw your left leg in towards your chest. Simultaneously straighten your right leg away, in line with your hip. With the same out breath, switch leg and arm positions. Repeat the action swiftly on both sides with the in breath. Repeat 8–10 times on each side. To finish, stay curled up, bend your knees into your chest. Keep your abdominals strong and lower your feet one by one, returning to the relaxation position.

Repeat 8–10 times on each side.

Double leg stretch STAGE 2

◆ GOOD FOR: Challenging muscles, stretching

The classical version of this exercise strengthens your abdominals and develops stamina and coordination, mobilizing your shoulders and hip joints.

Related exercise

Double leg stretch: stage 1 (page 67)

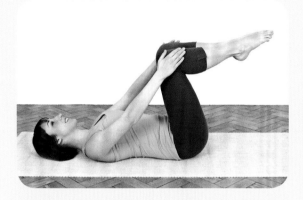

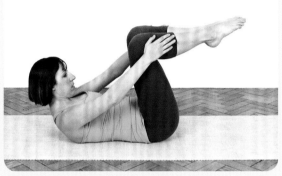

1 Start in the relaxation position with your pelvis and spine in neutral. Float your knees one by one into a double knee fold. Keep your feet connected with your toes softly pointed, and open your knees slightly. Lengthen your arms forward and place your hands lightly around your knees with the elbows soft.

2 Breathe in to prepare and lengthen your spine. As you breathe out, nod your nose forward and curl your upper body off the mat into a curl-up position.

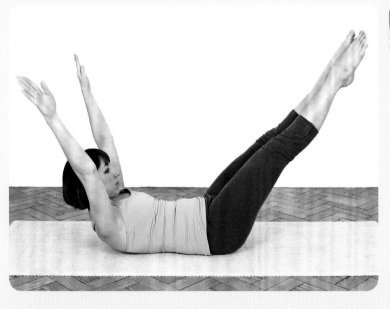

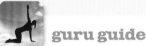

guru guide

• Make sure you do not lose your curl: maintain a strong connection with your abdominals.

• Focus your eyes forward rather than up to the ceiling.

3 Breathe in and press both legs away from your torso on a diagonal and draw your inner thighs together to bring your legs into Pilates stance. At the same time, lengthen your arms away in line with your ears. Maintain your curl up, with your eye focus towards your centre.

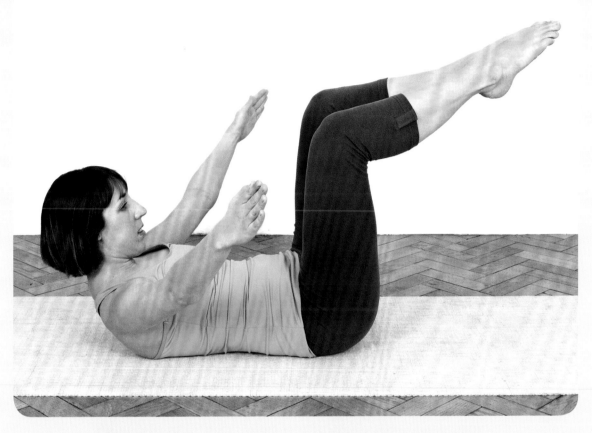

4 Breathe out to draw your legs back towards your body, keeping your heels connected as the knees open to shoulder width. Keep your abdominals strong and your spine and pelvis still as you move your limbs. Simultaneously, circle your arms out by your sides and take your hands around your knees.

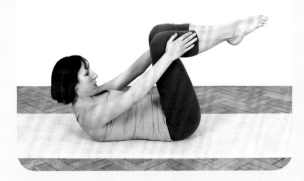

5 Rest your hands back around your knees into the start position as you breathe in. Repeat up to 10 times.

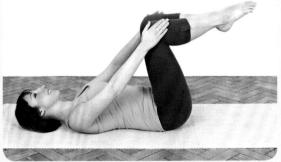

6 To finish, release your head and shoulders to the mat, and then gently float your feet back down, one by one, to end in the relaxation position.

Roll up

◆ GOOD FOR: Challenging muscles, stretching, spinal mobility

A classical Pilates exercise, this one requires great abdominal strength. It mobilizes your hips and spine and challenges your abdominals, aiming for fluidity and control in your movement.

Related exercises

Roll backs (pages 70–1)

Spine stretch forward (page 94)

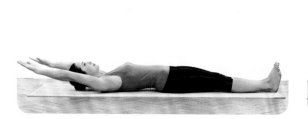

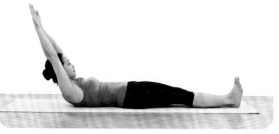

1 Lie on your back and find your neutral pelvis and spine. Connect your legs in parallel and flex your feet. Release your arms over your head in line with your ears, palms facing the ceiling and connecting your ribcage down into the floor. Engage your abdominals gently.

2 Breathe in, nod your chin to your chest and begin to curl your body from the mat, floating your arms in line with your ears.

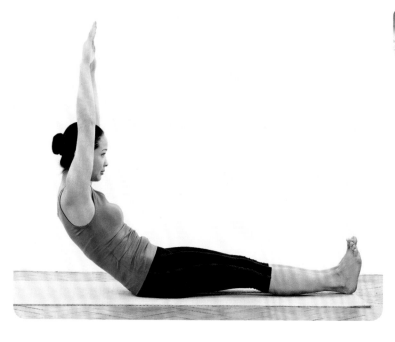

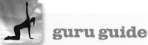 **guru guide**

• Make sure you use your abdominals to curl with control rather than any momentum created by throwing your torso forward. Keep the movement slow and even.

• Imagine length through your spine throughout the movement, trying not to allow your spine to feel compressed at any point. Keep your waist long.

3 Breathe out and continue to roll evenly through your spine, using your breath to control the movement.

Repeat up to **10 times,** allowing your **body** to find a **rhythm** and **flow** with the **movement.**

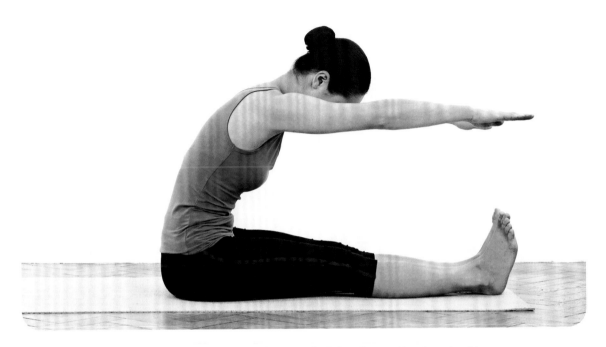

4 Curl up into a c-curve, reaching your arms forward over your toes and keeping them in line with your ears. Do not overreach. Breathe in, curl your tailbone under you and deepen your belly further as you begin to roll your pelvis back into the mat. Breathe out and keep rolling down using your abdominals to control the descent of your spine. Release your head and lengthen your arms behind you as you complete the exhalation. Repeat up to 10 times.

Making it easier

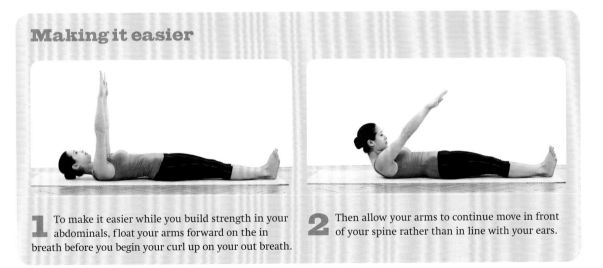

1 To make it easier while you build strength in your abdominals, float your arms forward on the in breath before you begin your curl up on your out breath.

2 Then allow your arms to continue move in front of your spine rather than in line with your ears.

Roll over

◆ GOOD FOR: Challenging muscles, stretching, spinal and joint mobility

This classical exercise is a dynamic version of a yoga posture, the plough. It develops abdominal strength and control, as well as challenging the leg and arm muscles. The focus here is on flowing movement, allowing the movement to continue using your breath and the strength of your muscles, not relying on momentum.

Repeat up to 4 times.

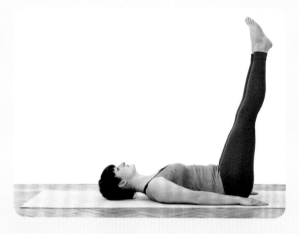

1 Lie on your back, float your knees to your chest, and extend your legs up to the ceiling, thighs connected and feet pointed. Lower your legs to where you can still maintain your neutral pelvis. Do not arch your back.

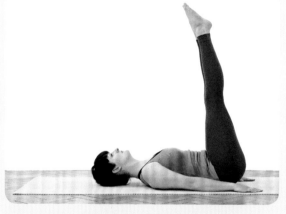

2 Breathe in as you deepen your abdominals and draw your legs in towards you, curling your tailbone under and beginning to lift your hips.

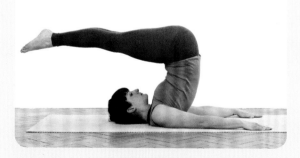

3 Breathe out and use your abdominals to roll your spine off the mat, floating your legs over your head until they are parallel to the floor. Don't roll too far into your neck, and keep your belly scooped.

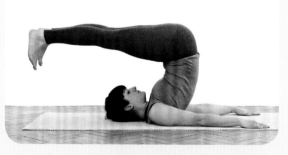

4 Breathe in, separate your legs to shoulder-width apart and flex your feet. Keep your spine long, do not allow it to dip but try to increase the flexion of your hips and draw your legs further towards your nose.

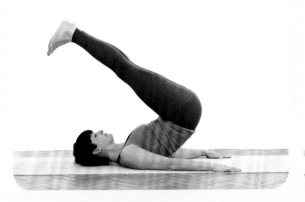

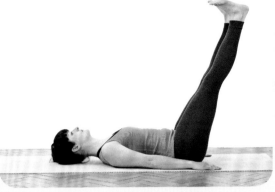

5 Breathe out and lower your hips to the mat. Articulate every bone of your spine. When your tailbone meets the mat, lower your legs towards the floor, keeping your abdominals strong so your back does not arch. Softly point your feet. Repeat up to 4 times.

6 Reverse the leg pattern. Have your legs shoulder-width apart and feet flexed. Breathe in, hinge at your hip and draw your legs in towards your body. Breathe out as you deepen the belly to roll your spine off the mat, pressing out through your heels. Roll over until your legs are parallel with the floor.

guru guide

• Try to avoid swinging your legs over your head with momentum: control the movement with your abdominals and use your breath to help you.

• Keep your arms connected to the ground from your shoulders to palms, and feel open across your chest. Keep your weight even on your arms.

• Roll in a straight line, central through your spine.

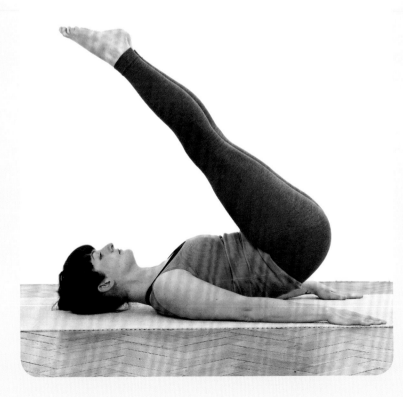

7 Breathe in, connect your inner thighs and point your feet. Breathe out and wheel your spine back down to the mat with control. When your tailbone reaches the mat, lower your legs towards the floor, keeping your spine in neutral. Open them to shoulder-width and flex your feet. Repeat up to 4 times. Return your legs directly to the ceiling, bend your knees and float your legs down to the mat, one by one, to the relaxation position.

Double leg kick

◆ GOOD FOR: Challenging muscles, stretching, spinal and joint mobility

This classical exercise works the hamstrings and buttocks, stretching the front of your thighs and strengthening your back muscles. This exercise requires working with all of the Pilates principles. The movement is precise and you need coordination and control, avoiding tension in your body by working the correct muscles.

Repeat up to 8 times, alternating your head position.

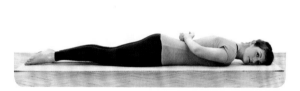

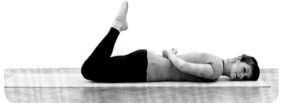

1 Align yourself on your front, pelvis and spine in neutral. Turn your face to the right and rest on your left cheek. Clasp your hands behind your back by sliding one hand into the palm of other, palms facing up (see below left). Place your hands as far up your back as you feel comfortable and release your elbows towards the mat. Your legs are together and in parallel. Connect to your centre.

2 Breathe in to prepare and lengthen your spine. Breathe out and kick both legs in towards your buttocks briskly 3 times. Keep your legs together and your pelvis level as you kick.

The hand position

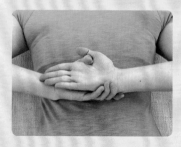

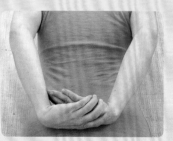

For step 1, lay one hand over the other and loop your thumbs. When you change the side that you face to, alternate which hand is on top.

For step 3, straighten your arms, and turn your palms to face your back as you loop your thumbs together and open your chest.

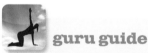

guru guide

• Keep your abdominals strong throughout.

• Try not to arch your back: stay lengthened and controlled.

• Control the movement back to the mat rather than letting your body collapse.

Making it harder

In step 3, as you breathe in and stretch your legs, lengthen your feet slightly from the floor – your abdominals will have to work harder to keep your spine stable.

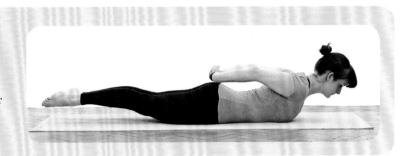

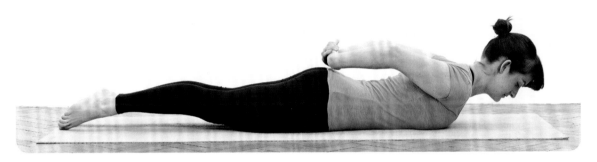

3 Breathe in and stretch your legs long behind you. Simultaneously begin to lift your spine, turning your head so the eye focus is down to the floor. The upper spine extends as you open your chest. Straighten your arms, looping your thumbs together (see hand position box) and turn your palms to face your back. Reach your arms slightly away from your buttocks. Make sure your abdominals are lifted and your neck and spine stay long. Your eye focus is now forward.

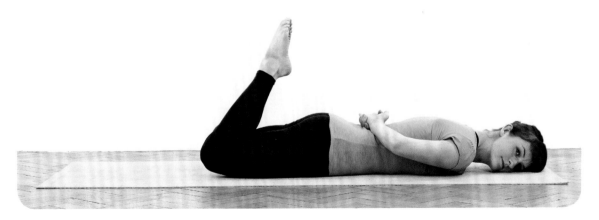

4 Breathe out and release your body back to the floor. Kick your legs dynamically 3 times in towards your buttocks once more as you return your spine to the mat and bring your arms into the mid-back to start again. Turn your face to the left and repeat up to 8 times, alternating your head position.

Swan dive

◆ GOOD FOR: Challenging muscles, spinal mobility

This is a beautiful exercise from Joe Pilates' classical repertoire. A strengthening and invigorating exercise, it requires great spinal and abdominal strength and encourages openness in the front of your body and legs.

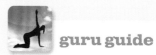

guru guide

• Feel that your spine is stable and does not change its shape with the rocking motion.

• Keep your abdominals very strong and spine stable and think about maintaining length at all times.

• Keep your head in line with your spine and shoulders away from your ears.

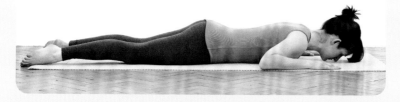

1 Lie on your front with your spine and pelvis in neutral. Position your legs slightly wider than hip-width apart and turned out from the hip. Place your hands down in line with your ears, slightly wider than your shoulders, elbows bent. Gently stabilize and lengthen your spine by drawing in your abdominals.

> ### Related exercises
>
> Cobra (page 104)
>
> Double leg lifts (page 105)

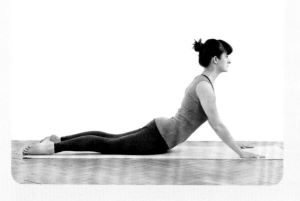

2 Breathe in and move into cobra, lengthening your spine in extension. Allow your arms to straighten as your spine reaches its full length, pelvis lifted and supported by your abdominals.

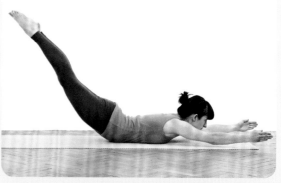

3 Extend your arms forward in line with your ears, palms facing in. You will rock forward onto your ribcage. Lengthen your legs high behind you. Feel energy reaching out through your feet and an openness around your hip joints. Keep your abdominals strong.

Use your momentum for 5–6 rocks.

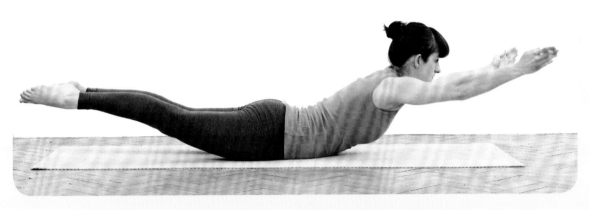

4 Breathe in and rock back using your own momentum. Your legs reach down towards the floor as your torso lifts high. Keep your legs straight and actively reaching away through the movement at all times, and remember to keep your abdominal muscles strong.

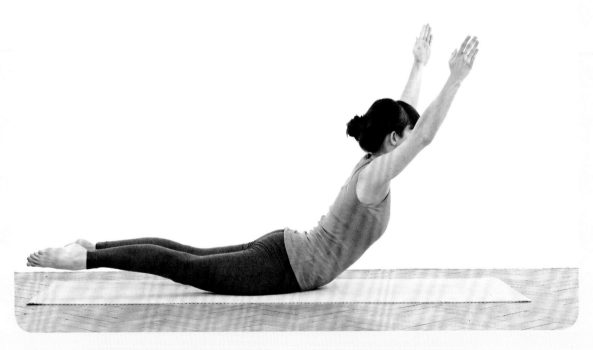

5 Keep reaching forward through your fingertips and feel length throughout your whole body. Use your momentum for 5–6 rocks. To finish the swan dive, bring your hands down, and press back into the rest position to allow your back to release in a counterpose.

Swimming

◆ GOOD FOR: Challenging muscles, spinal and joint mobility

A dynamic, classical Pilates exercise, swimming develops awareness of symmetry and opposition in the body, working each side of your body equally, with stability and control. It also helps develops stamina and strength in your upper back, shoulders and buttocks.

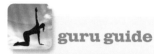

guru guide

• Keep your legs straight, dynamically reaching away from your torso. Your pelvis should remain still and grounded into the mat.

• Do not overreach your arms, keep your neck long.

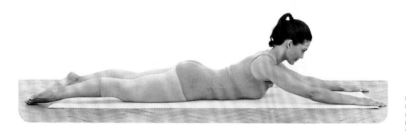

1 Align yourself on your front, arms lengthened out in front of you at slightly wider than shoulder-width apart, and legs released away, hip-width apart and in parallel. Open your throat to lift your head and chest slightly from the mat, extending your upper spine and engaging your abdominals. Keep your palms connected to the floor and shoulders softly connected to your body. Keep your eye focus forward.

Related exercises

Table top (pages 72–3)

Prone leg lifts (page 75)

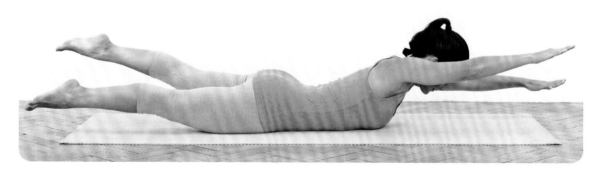

2 Breathe in to prepare and lengthen your spine. Breathe out, scoop your belly as you lengthen and lift one arm off the floor and reach the opposite leg away behind you. Breathe in, and lower and lift opposite arms and legs in a swift beating motion, for a count of 5. Breathe out for a count of 5 and continue to beat your arms and legs. Begin slowly and pick up speed, but don't lose control. After up to 10 breaths, lower your arms and legs to the mat, and press yourself into the rest position (see page 38) to release your spine and neck.

Hinge back (thigh stretch)

◆ GOOD FOR: Challenging muscles, stretching, joint mobility

This exercise tones your buttocks and challenges your powerhouse and the ability to move your body as one connected unit. It stretches your thighs and focuses on control and length of your spine.

Repeat up to 8 times.

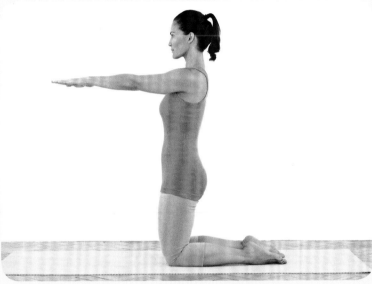

1 Kneel upright with your legs hip-width apart. Extend your arms in front of you at shoulder height, with palms facing down. Reach your fingers forward and think of lengthening up through the crown of your head before you begin to move.

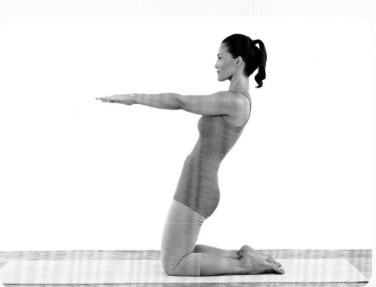

2 Breathe in to prepare and lengthen the back of your neck. Breathe out and begin to hinge back, moving your body in a straight line from your knees to the crown of your head. Breathe in to hold the position, squeezing your buttocks and feeling the front of your thighs opening. Breathe out and, using your belly and bottom, hinge forward in one piece back to the upright position. Repeat up to 8 times.

Push ups from standing

◆ GOOD FOR: Challenging muscles, stretching, joint mobility

This is a challenging exercise requiring great strength, control and stability. It strengthens your arms and shoulders, as well as your abdominals.

Repeat up to 3 times.

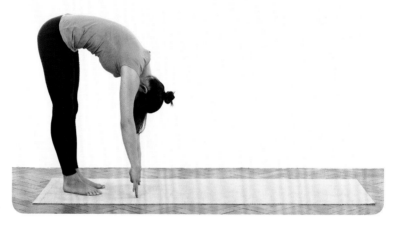

2 Breathe in, lengthen your spine and connect to your centre. Nod your chin and begin to lower your arms, curling your upper body and rolling your spine down until your hands reach the mat.

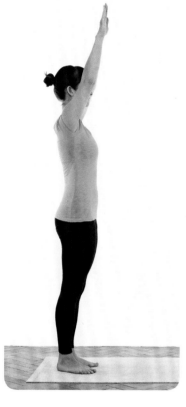

1 Stand in Pilates stance, spine in neutral. Raise your arms directly above your head, in line with your ears and with palms facing forward.

Related exercises

Roll downs (pages 46–7)

Cat to down dog (pages 112–13)

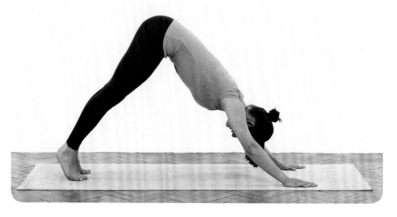

3 Breathe out and begin to walk your hands out into a plank position, with your hands directly underneath your shoulders, and pelvis and spine in neutral.

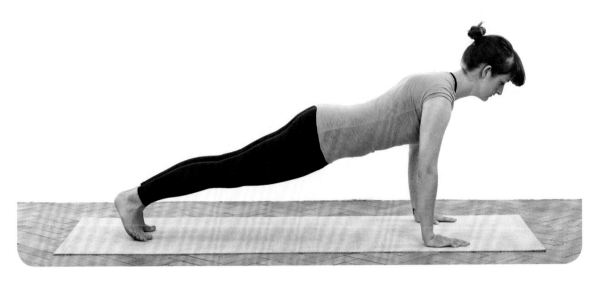

4 Once you are in plank, ensure that your heels are still connected and your inner thighs working. Stay in one long line from the crown of your head to your heels. Keep your buttocks working and inner thighs connected.

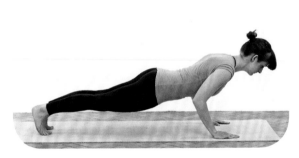

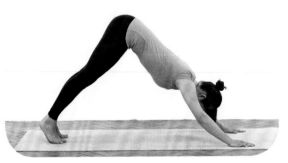

5 Breathe in and bend your elbows in towards your waist – not out to the side. Lower your body in a straight line towards the floor. Breathe out and straighten your elbows, lifting the body in one connected unit back to the plank position. Repeat this push up 3 times.

6 Breathe in, press your heels back and use your abdominals to lift your bottom towards the ceiling into a down dog position, nodding your chin to your chest. Breathe out and to walk your hands back towards your feet, as in step 2. Breathe in and restack your spine and raise your arms above your head as in step 1. Repeat up to 3 times.

Making it easier

If you find it too difficult to keep your elbows near your body when doing the push up, build up your strength by allowing them to open outwards.

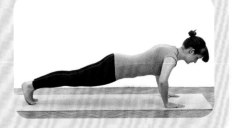

guru guide

• As you press down in step 5, keep your abdominals strong and avoid arching your back.

• When restacking your spine to come back up, use your abdominals.

advanced exercises 133

Kneeling side kicks

◆ GOOD FOR: Challenging muscles, joint mobility

From the classical mat, this dynamic exercise challenges your balance and spinal stability, mobilizing your hips as you kick with strength and rhythm.

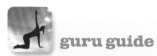

guru guide

• Keep your eye focus forward and neck in line with your spine.

• Control the movement: if you cannot swing your leg without moving your torso, practise easier leg kicks (pages 78–9) to strengthen your core before moving on to this exercise.

Repeat up to 8 times on each leg.

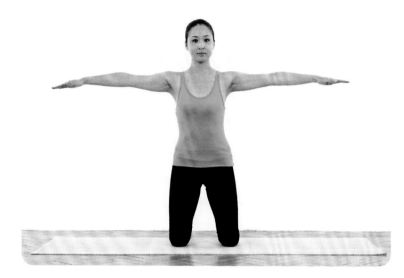

1 Kneel upright and raise both arms at shoulder height.

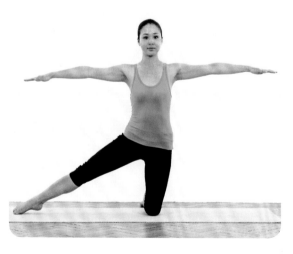

2 Extend your right leg directly out to the side in line with your body, toes softly pointed.

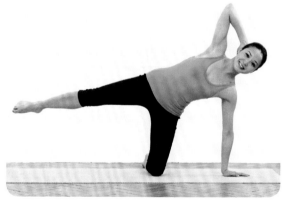

3 With strong abdominals, lengthen your body to the left, placing your left hand on the mat directly under your shoulder, with your arm straight. Take your right hand behind your head. Deepen your abdominals to raise your right leg in line with your pelvis, parallel to the mat.

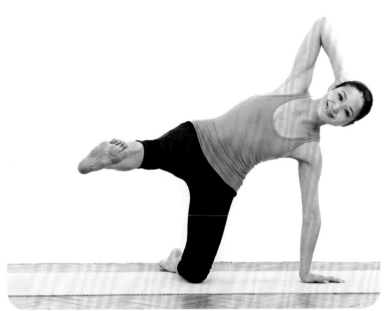

4 Breathe in wide and full and engage your centre to kick your right leg to the front, without allowing your body to rock forward or back.

Making it easier

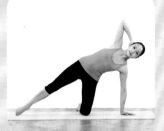

1 If swinging your leg forward is too challenging for your balance, practise holding this position with leg lifts to build your strength. When you are able to control this leg lift with no movement of your torso, you can attempt the forward leg kicks. Assume the starting position as in steps 1–3, opposite, leaving the foot of your left leg on the floor.

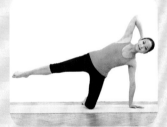

2 Instead of kicking your leg forward, lift it to hip height with your out breath, then lower. Repeat 8 times, and then move to the other side.

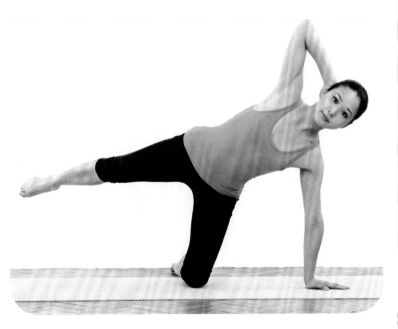

5 Breathe out and swing your leg back, lengthening it slightly behind the body to open your hip, but without allowing your back to arch. Stay strong and stable with your abdominals and long in the waist. Repeat up to 8 times with this leg, then return to step 1 and repeat with the other leg.

Related exercises

Side-lying leg kicks (pages 78–9)

advanced exercises **135**

Climb a tree

◆ GOOD FOR: Challenging muscles, stretching, joint mobility

This exercise is wonderful for highlighting weaknesses of one side of your body over the other together with any postural misalignments. It is a challenging abdominal workout, requiring smooth movement and focuses on your coordination and control.

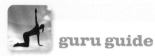

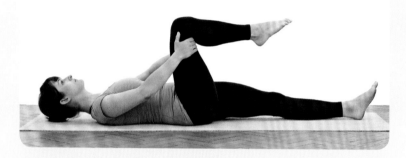

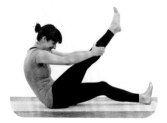

1 Lie in the relaxation position with your left leg straight and lengthened, foot softly pointed, and your right leg bent in towards your body. Find your neutral spine and pelvis and soften your shoulders. Take your hands behind your right thigh.

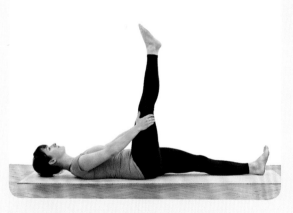

2 Breathe in to draw your abdominals in as you extend your right leg towards the ceiling.

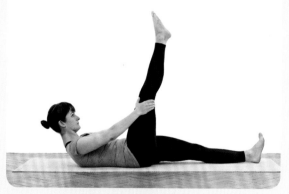

3 Breathe out, nod your chin to your chest and curl up as you walk your hands up your leg towards your ankle. Do not drag yourself up with your hands, use your abdominals. Keep your chest open and abdominals strong.

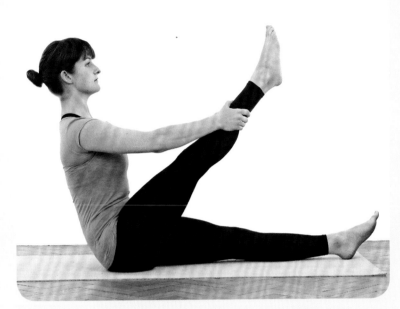

Related exercise
Scissors (pages 96–7)

Repeat up to 5 times on each leg.

4 As you approach your ankle, your leg will lengthen away as your spine moves, but keep it as lifted as possible and do not allow it to drop to the floor. Keep your left leg heavy and stable. Breathe in to lift through your spine at the top.

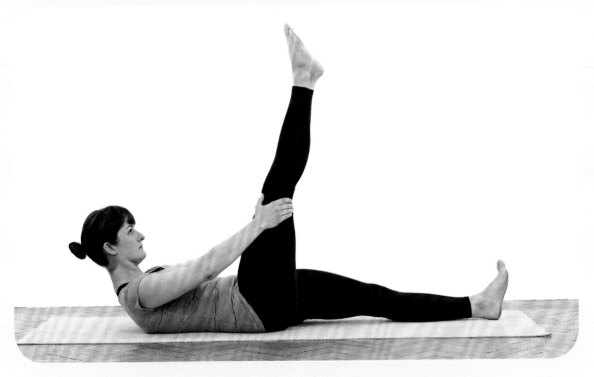

5 As you breathe out, begin to lower your spine slowly, walking your hands down your leg, and control the release of your spine down to the mat with your abdominals. Repeat up to 5 times on one leg, then repeat on the other. To finish, float your feet back to the floor into relaxation position.

The teaser

◆ GOOD FOR: Challenging muscles, spinal and joint mobility

The ultimate abdominal challenge, legend has it that Joe Pilates would dangle a $50 note in front of his clients with this exercise to see if they were able to reach up and grab it, hence the name. This exercise requires great strength, control and balance. When you can perform the half teaser (see pages 102–3) with control, you are ready to move on to this advanced version.

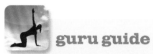

guru guide

• Stay lengthened in your spine throughout: deeply engage your abdominals and do not allow your spine to curl underneath and shoulders to hunch forward. Stay lifted and open.

• Try not to grip across the front of your hips: instead, use your inner thigh connection and pelvic floor for strength.

Related exercise

The half teaser (pages 102–3)

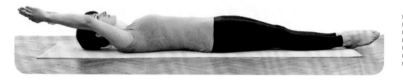

1 Lie on your back, with spine and pelvis in neutral. Lengthen your arms above your head, in line with your ears, palms facing up, and release your legs out in line with your body and with the inner thighs connected in Pilates stance.

Repeat up to 5 times.

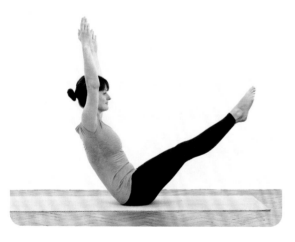

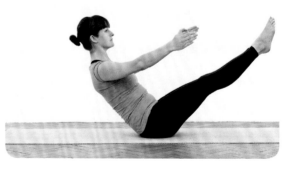

2 Breathe in to prepare and lengthen your spine. Breathe out as you nod your chin forward and begin to curl your spine, keeping your arms level with your ears. Simultaneously, lift both legs to create a letter 'V'.

3 Reach your fingers forward towards your feet, keeping your arms parallel with your legs.

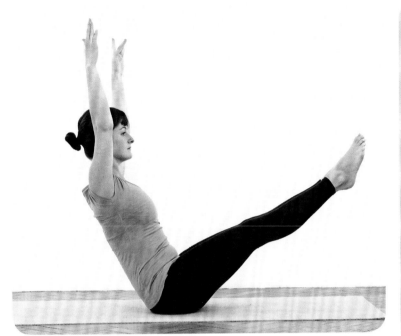

Making it harder

To further work your abdominal muscles, once you are in position in step 4, lower your legs a little further towards the ground, keeping your spine stable, chest lifted and abdominals strong. Then draw your legs back up towards you, back into the 'V' position and continue with step 5.

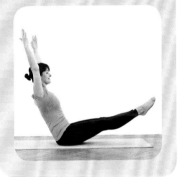

4 Breathe in and, staying very strong and lifted with the upper body and keeping your legs controlled, lengthen your arms above your head in line with your ears once more. Keep your eye focus forward and chest lifted.

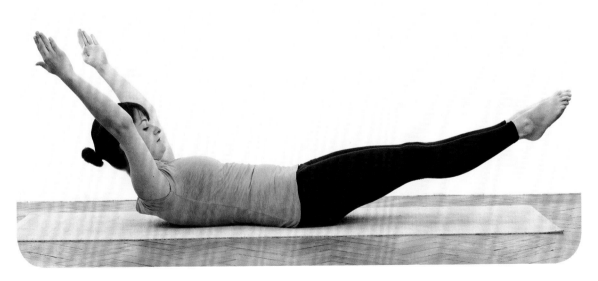

5 Breathe out and begin to roll your pelvis underneath you, controlling the descent of your upper body and legs simultaneously. Keep your arms lengthened above your head as you release your spine. Then release your body and legs down with an in breath. Repeat up to 5 times.

Criss cross

◆ GOOD FOR: Challenging muscles, stretching, spinal and joint mobility

One of the most challenging abdominal exercises, you will really feel the burn after this one. This exercise develops both strength and stamina, requiring control and coordination.

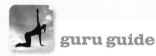

guru guide

• The movement of the twist should come from your ribcage and not your elbows.

• Stay long on both sides of your waist throughout the exercise.

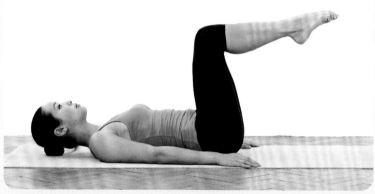

Related exercise

Obliques (pages 58–9)

1 Lie in your relaxation position, spine and pelvis in neutral. Float both knees into your chest.

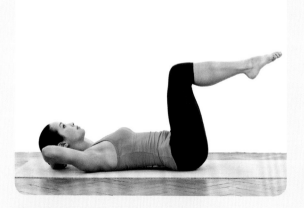

2 Clasp your hands behind your head with your elbows in your peripheral vision.

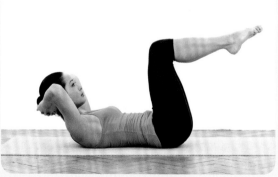

3 Connect to your powerhouse and curl up towards your knees. Keep your abdominals scooped and tailbone heavy.

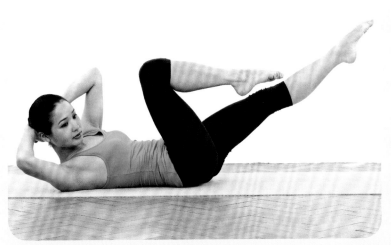

Repeat up to
8 times
to each side.

4 Breathe in wide and full into your back, keeping your belly engaged. Breathe out as you lengthen and reach your left leg away from you, pressing your foot away with resistance as if you are pressing a pedal. Simultaneously, twist your body towards your right bent leg, drawing your knee further in towards you, using your abdominals.

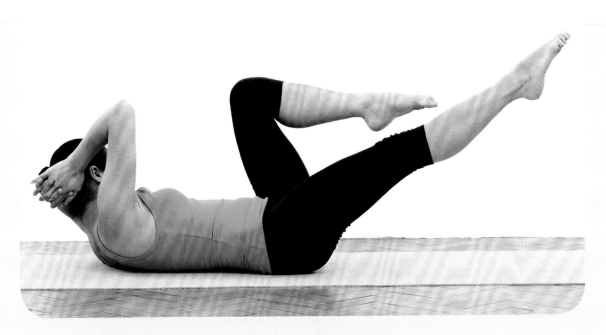

5 Breathe in to draw your left leg back towards you and return your torso to the centre. Breathe out and twist across to the left, extending your right leg away. Maintain the height of your curl as you twist your ribcage, and stay anchored across your hips. Repeat up to 8 times to each side.

advanced exercises 141

Side plank: star

◆ GOOD FOR: Challenging muscles, joint mobility

This exercise challenges your core muscles and stability, requiring you to move with control, always lengthening your limbs from a strong centre. It is a great way to build strength and balance.

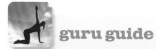

guru guide

• For the main exercise, rest on the edge of one foot. If you need to, you can bring your other foot down in front for balance.

• Engage your abdominals strongly throughout to ensure no movement of your spine. Always aim for free movement of your limbs from a stable centre.

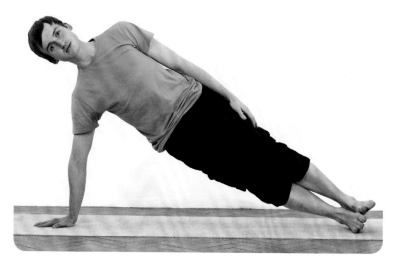

1 Sit on your hip, with your legs folded to one side, heels in line with your bottom, feet stacked on top of each other. Place your arm out by your side, slightly wider than your shoulder. Breathe in to prepare and lengthen your spine. As you breathe out, initiate your abdominals to press yourself into a side plank, lifting up with the hips. Bring your body into one long line, squeezing your inner thighs and abdominals.

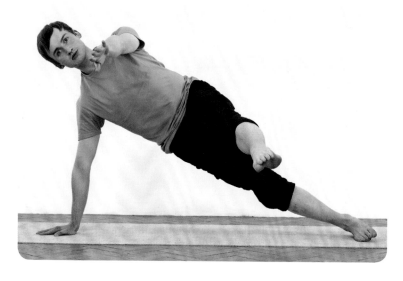

2 Breathe in to balance and lengthen. As you breathe out, swing your top leg forward from your hip, taking your top arm forward at the same time. Lengthen your limbs only as far as you can without disturbing your neutral pelvis and spine – no swinging of the spine to follow the limbs. Breathe in to return your arm and leg to the central side plank position.

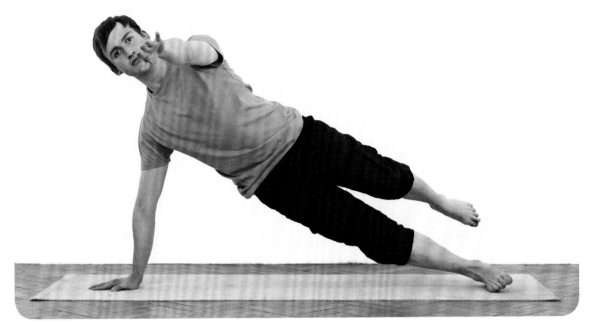

3 Breathe out and lengthen your top leg back and take your top arm forward. Feel your hip opening but do not allow your back to arch, and keep your abdominals strong to stabilize the spine. Feel you are lengthening your arm and leg in opposition from fingertips to toes. Breathe in to return your arm and leg to the central side plank position. Repeat up to 5 times, alternating front and back. To finish, lower to the mat with control. Repeat the exercise on the other side.

Making it easier

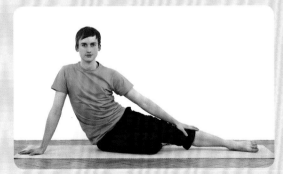

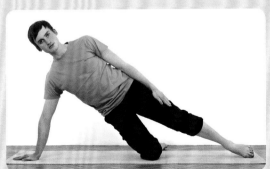

1 If you need assistance with the balance while you build strength, rest your bottom knee on the floor to give you more support.

2 Push up into the side plank, as before, but keeping your bottom knee on the floor. Move your arms and legs as in the main exercise.

Rowing

◆ GOOD FOR: Challenging muscles, stretching, joint mobility

Another demanding exercise adapted from Joe Pilates'
apparatus repertoire. This exercise requires great
strength, control and coordination.

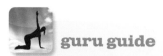

guru guide

• Keep those abdominals
working throughout.

• Stay energized: feel that you are
anchored into the mat through
your heels, legs and pelvis, but
light and lifted through the crown
of your head.

• Try to avoid gripping in the
front of your hips. Instead, use
your buttocks, pelvic floor and
inner thighs.

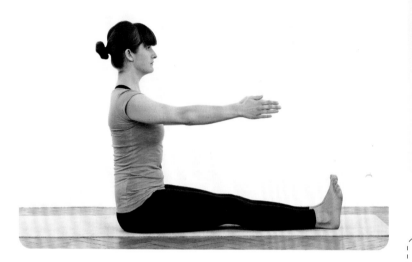

1 Sit upright, directly on your sitting bones with your legs parallel and
extended in front of you, feet flexed. Release your arms in front of you,
in line with your shoulders and with palms facing each other. Breathe in
wide and full to prepare and lengthen your spine. Lengthen your ribcage
away from your hips and sit tall.

Related exercises

C-curve (page 39)

Spine stretch forward
(page 94)

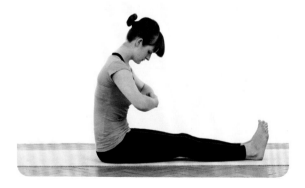

2 Breathe out and lift your pelvic floor, deepening
your abdominal connection. Breathe in and curl your
tailbone beneath you to start to roll into a c-curve. At the
same time, bring your hands into fists with your knuckles
together near your breastbone, elbows out to the sides.

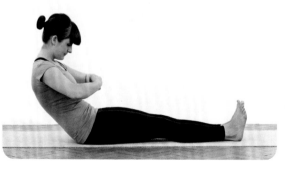

3 Continue to roll back until you can no longer
control the movement with your abdominals. Keep
your chest open, and neck long and eye focus forward.
Keep your legs on the floor and feet flexed, pressing
energy out through your heels.

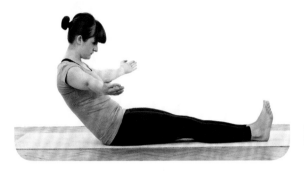

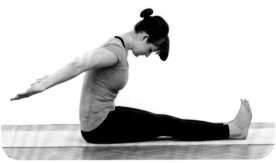

4 Breathe out and extend your hands out to the sides, releasing your fingers long as you lengthen your arms out in line with your shoulders, palms facing forward. Head and body stay stable and still. When your arms are extended, rotate your palms to face the floor.

5 Breathe in and begin to roll back up through your spine, using your belly. At the same time, press your hands behind you, as if you are pushing through water like oars. Rotate your wrists so your palms face the ceiling. Your belly is lifted and your eye focus towards your knees.

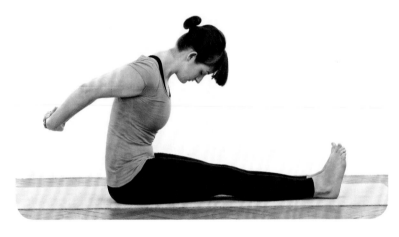

Repeat up to 5 times.

6 Clasp your hands together and reach your arms back behind you, lifting out towards the ceiling. Deepen your bend forward but keep your abdominals strong and do not collapse your chest.

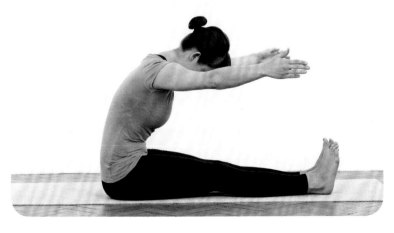

7 Breathe out and release your hands with control, beginning to circle your arms forward, rotating your palms down. Reach your arms all the way to your toes. Restack your spine into your sitting start position, smoothly and with control. Breathe in and repeat up to 5 times.

advanced exercises 145

Seal

◆ GOOD FOR: Challenging muscles, spinal and joint mobility

This is a dynamic way to strengthen your abdominals and the stability of your c-curve. Playful and demanding, it massages the spine and focuses on coordinating the rhythm of your breath with your movement.

Related exercise

Rolling like a ball (page 89)

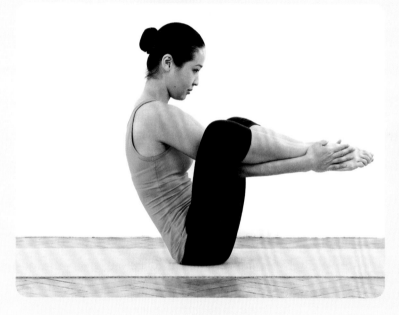

1 Make sure there is room on your mat to roll back. Sit in your c-curve, tailbone curled under and long in your spine, abdominals lifted. Bend your knees in and open your hip joints to bring the soles of your feet together. Thread your hands between your knees and take hold of the outside of your ankles. Tip back and find your balance, maintaining this position. Breathe out to deepen your abdominals and prepare for rolling back.

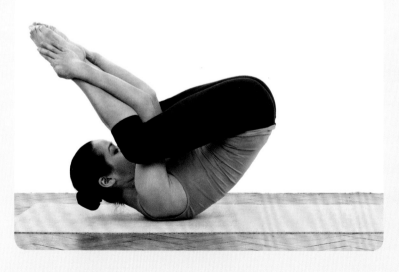

2 Breathe in and roll back smoothly, maintaining the curved shape of your spine and leg position, allowing your tailbone to roll up to the ceiling. Keep your head tucked in, chin to chest, and stay strong in the abdominals. Balance briefly here, and clap the soles of your feet together 3 times (see above right), moving from your hip joint.

guru guide

• Make sure you coordinate the movement to your breath, and keep your belly scooped and your waist long throughout.

• The foot clap (see right) is a way of mobilizing your hip joints. Make each clap a controlled movement, precisely opening your hips and closing them as you beat your feet together.

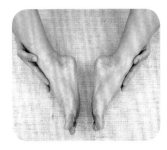

Repeat up to
10 times.

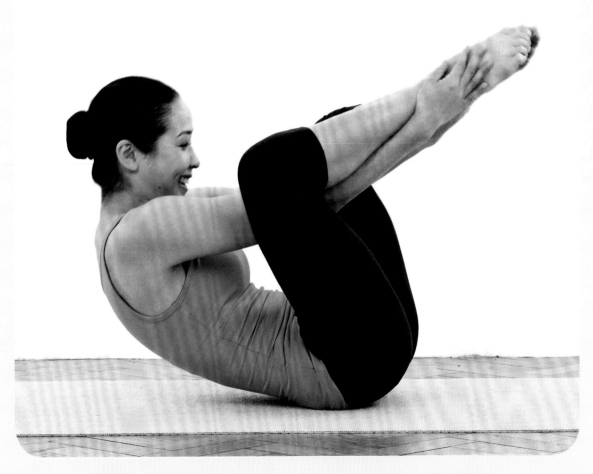

3 Breathe out and rock back onto your tailbone, making sure you do not lose the shape of your spine and legs. Balance and pause at the top position and clap your feet once more. Breathe in to roll back and clap your feet. Place both feet back onto the floor to finish. Repeat up to 10 times.

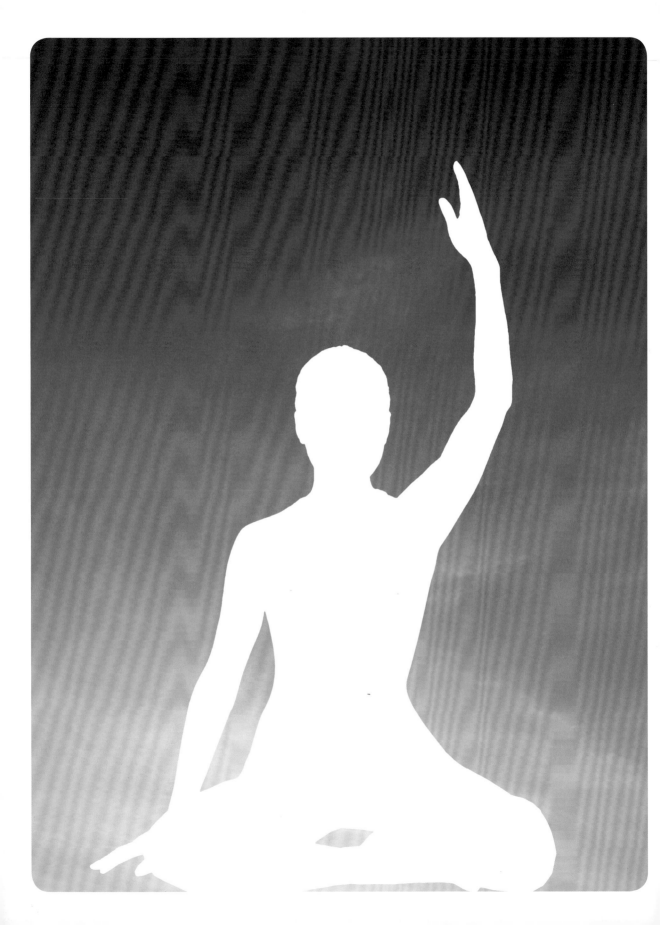

Pilates sessions

In this section you look at how to create your own routines. All Pilates workouts need to be balanced and combine the right amount of challenge and relaxation. Here you find out what elements you should include in each workout and how best to structure your routine for an effective, demanding and fun workout that will make your practice enjoyable and never boring.

Structuring your workouts

The structure of your Pilates workouts should follow a certain order: first you need to warm up, moving on to challenging your muscles and stretching all muscle groups in the core of your workout, and finishing with a cool down. Before beginning the core section (see overleaf), ensure you warm up and sufficiently prepare your body, and then allow your body time to cool down at the end.

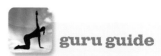

guru guide

• Never exercise if you are feeling unwell or if you have been drinking alcohol.

• Always warm up and cool down.

Warming up and cooling down

In each workout first warm up your muscles to ensure they are ready to be challenged. Never skip the warm up as it encourages blood supply to your muscles and prepares your body, helping to prevent injuries, and aches or pains.

First mobilize your spine. Make sure you spend at least 2 or 3 minutes at the start of your workout with gentle exercises from the basics and beginner levels (see below). These exercises will also encourage you to focus on your breath and connect your mind to your body. Then warm up your joints, with exercises such as those listed opposite below.

The warm-up section of your workout should include at least five or six different exercises, and take up to 10 minutes.

Warming up exercises

These exercises are ideal for warming up before moving onto the core of a workout. For others, see the 'Good for' line at the top of each exercise.

MOBILIZING YOUR SPINE

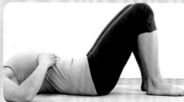

Pelvic clocks and tilts (page 27)

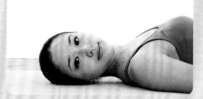

Neck rolls (page 33)

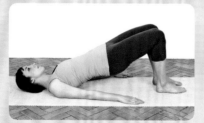

Spine curls (page 34)

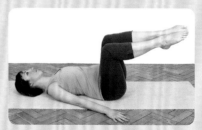

Hip rolls (pages 60–1)

Every workout should also include a cool down period of up to 10 minutes at the end. Through cool down exercises (see below) you give your body a chance to slow down after the intensity of the challenging section, recover, and incorporate some relaxation so that your workout leaves you feeling refreshed in body and mind.

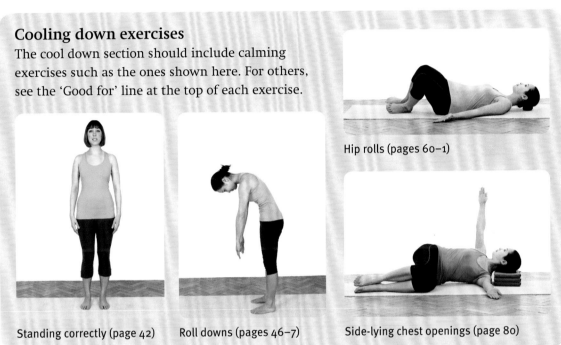

Cooling down exercises

The cool down section should include calming exercises such as the ones shown here. For others, see the 'Good for' line at the top of each exercise.

Hip rolls (pages 60–1)

Standing correctly (page 42)

Roll downs (pages 46–7)

Side-lying chest openings (page 80)

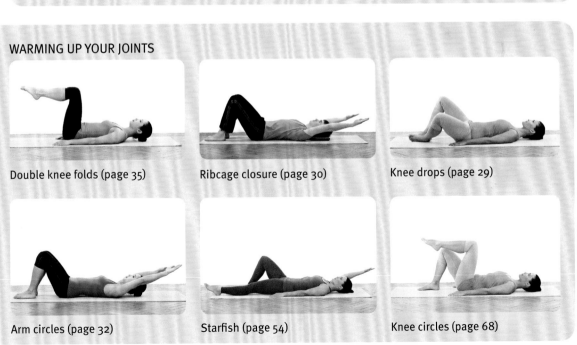

WARMING UP YOUR JOINTS

Double knee folds (page 35)

Ribcage closure (page 30)

Knee drops (page 29)

Arm circles (page 32)

Starfish (page 54)

Knee circles (page 68)

The core of your workouts

The focus of your Pilates workouts should be equally on your whole body and using all planes of movement of the spine, as shown on page 18. At the same time include sufficient variety of exercises so that your muscles are challenged and your body stretched. A balanced workout will include all of these components and work your whole body evenly, ensuring that your spine has been fully mobilized and the muscles on the front and back of your body have been equally strengthened and released.

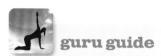

guru guide

• In the pages that follow choose from various workouts created to suit different times and moods. Use them as a template to create your own challenges according to how your body is feeling, different areas you want to focus on and how hard you want to work.

Challenging your muscles

Always begin with a lower level of challenge and gradually layer on the difficulty, speed and complexity (see examples below).

Ensure you try to challenge all muscle groups by incorporating all movements of the spine and on all planes of movement: include at least one exercise lying on your back, on your front, side-lying and four-point kneeling. This part forms the main body of your workout – up to 45 minutes for an hour's workout. You can intersperse very challenging exercises with easier ones, to give your body a rest and ensure you don't become fatigued.

Challenging muscles

The exercises given here are examples that challenge your muscles to different degrees. Use the 'Good for' line at the top of each exercise to choose others that suit you and your ability.

LOWER LEVEL

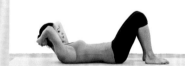

Curl ups (pages 56–7)

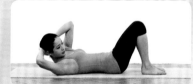

Obliques (pages 58–9)

HIGHER LEVEL

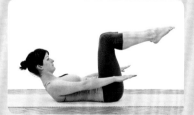

The hundred (pages 88 and 118)

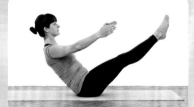

The teaser (pages 138–9)

Stretching your body

Throughout each workout you should include some stretches, too, which fill the dual role of giving your body some breathing space between challenging exercises, and allowing your muscles to stretch safely while they are warm.

Stretch muscles after you've worked them to give them a chance to repair and lessen the chance of horrible muscle ache in the days after your workout. It is also important to regularly stretch out from daily life to redress muscle imbalances. Choose stretches that are dynamic as well as more static stretches (see below). When stretching, ensure you are completely relaxed and in perfect alignment (a mirror can be helpful), and that you never overstretch: it should feel like a lengthening of the muscle and release of tension, not a painful strain.

Stretching out

The exercises given here are examples that stretch your body both dynamically and statically. Use the 'Good for' line at the top of each exercise to choose others that suit you and your ability. You can also incorporate stretches into your cool down (see page 151).

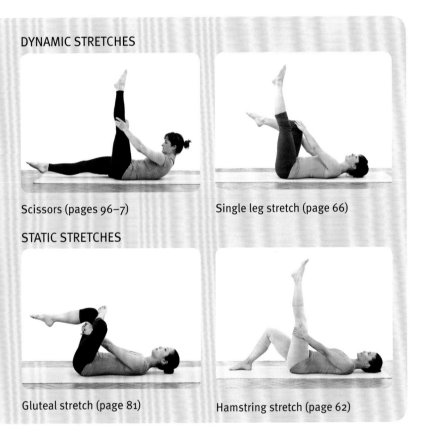

DYNAMIC STRETCHES

Scissors (pages 96–7)

Single leg stretch (page 66)

STATIC STRETCHES

Gluteal stretch (page 81)

Hamstring stretch (page 62)

Know your level

Before you attempt the intermediate or advanced level of an exercise, make sure you feel confident with the beginner's level. If you have any difficulty starting a higher-level exercise, revisit the earlier version (the page numbers are given on the appropriate exercises) and focus on gradually increasing the repetitions, to improve your stamina and confidence. Then have another go.

Pilates for posture

This is where Pilates comes into its own. Every Pilates exercise encourages you to learn about your alignment and be aware of how you carry yourself day to day, so that you can begin to coax your body into better balance.

Start with a few minutes of deep breathing (page 20). Ensure you are standing correctly (page 42), then continue with your choice of routine. Cool down in the rest position (page 38) and, if you have time, include other cool down exercises (page 151).

15-minute session

1 Rising on toes + floating arms (page 45)

2 Roll downs (pages 46–7)

3 Pec stretch (page 31)

4 Starfish (page 54)

5 Spine curls (page 34)

6 Obliques (page 58)

7 Dart (page 74)

8 Cat (page 41)

9 Table top (pages 72–3)

30-minute session

1 Rising on toes + floating arms (page 45)

2 Roll downs (pages 46–7)

3 Pec stretch (page 31)

4 Starfish (page 54)

5 Spine curls (page 34)

6 Obliques (page 58)

7 Hamstring stretch (page 62)

8 Hip flexor stretch (page 63)

9 The hundred: stage 1 (page 65)

10 Rolling like a ball (page 89)

11 Single leg stretch: stage 1 (page 66)

12 Dart (page 74)

13 Cat (page 41)

14 Table top (pages 72–3)

15 Thread the needle (page 110)

Related exercises for greater impact

Waist twist	Saw (pages 114–15)
Spine curls	Spine curls: progression (pages 100–1)
The hundred	Stages 2/3 (pages 88/118)
Single leg stretch	Stages 2/3 (pages 92–3/117)

guru guide

• Make sure you focus particularly on the precision of your movement and positioning throughout.

30-minute session

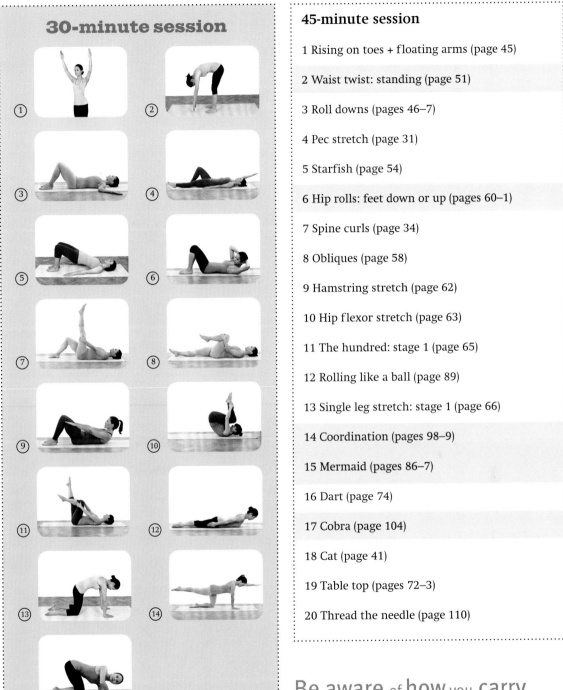

45-minute session

1 Rising on toes + floating arms (page 45)

2 Waist twist: standing (page 51)

3 Roll downs (pages 46–7)

4 Pec stretch (page 31)

5 Starfish (page 54)

6 Hip rolls: feet down or up (pages 60–1)

7 Spine curls (page 34)

8 Obliques (page 58)

9 Hamstring stretch (page 62)

10 Hip flexor stretch (page 63)

11 The hundred: stage 1 (page 65)

12 Rolling like a ball (page 89)

13 Single leg stretch: stage 1 (page 66)

14 Coordination (pages 98–9)

15 Mermaid (pages 86–7)

16 Dart (page 74)

17 Cobra (page 104)

18 Cat (page 41)

19 Table top (pages 72–3)

20 Thread the needle (page 110)

Be aware of how you carry yourself day to day.

Pilates for abdominals

If what you're after is a flat stomach, this is the workout for you. All Pilates exercises work the abdominals, but this routine particularly targets the deep stabilizing muscles around your spine and the oblique muscles of your waist, toning your whole abdominal area.

Start with a few minutes of deep breathing in the relaxation position (pages 20 and 24), then continue with your choice of routine. Cool down with roll downs (pages 46–7) and, if you have time, include other cool down exercises (page 151).

15-minute session

1 Pelvic clocks and tilts (page 27)

2 Spine curls (page 34)

3 Hip rolls: feet down or up (pages 60–1)

4 Curl ups (page 56)

5 The hundred: stage 1 (page 65)

6 Single leg stretch: stage 1 (page 66)

7 Double leg stretch: stage 1 (page 67)

8 Mermaid (pages 86–7)

9 Dart with arm circles (pages 106–7)

10 Torpedo (pages 108–9)

30-minute session

1 Pelvic clocks and tilts (page 27)

2 Spine curls (page 34)

3 Hip rolls: feet down or up (pages 60–1)

4 Curl ups (page 56)

5 Obliques with leg slide (page 59)

6 The hundred: stage 1 (page 65)

7 Rolling like a ball (page 89)

8 Single leg stretch: stage 1 (page 66)

9 Double leg stretch: stage 1 (page 67)

10 Mermaid (pages 86–7)

11 Scissors (pages 96–7)

12 Criss cross (pages 140–1)

13 Dart with arm circles (pages 106–7)

14 Torpedo (pages 108–9)

Related exercises for greater impact

Spine curls	Spine curls: progression (pages 100–1)	Single leg stretch	Stages 2/3 (pages 92–3/117)
The hundred	Stages 2/3 (pages 88/118)	Double leg stretch	Stage 2 (pages 120–1)

guru guide

• Focus on perfecting the centring techniques from page 26 to make sure you are engaging your muscles correctly. You will definitely feel the burn, but will soon see the amazing results.

30-minute session

① ②

③ ④

⑤ ⑥

⑦ ⑧

⑨ ⑩

⑪ ⑫

⑬ ⑭

45-minute session

1 Pelvic clocks and tilts (page 27)

2 Spine curls (page 34)

3 Hip rolls: feet down or up (pages 60–1)

4 Curl ups (page 56)

5 Obliques with leg slide (page 59)

6 The hundred: stage 1 (page 65)

7 Roll up (pages 122–3)

8 Rolling like a ball (page 89)

9 Single leg stretch: stage 1 (page 66)

10 Double leg stretch: stage 1 (page 67)

11 Mermaid (pages 86–7)

12 Scissors (pages 96–7)

13 Criss cross (pages 140–1)

14 Dart with arm circles (pages 106–7)

15 Swan dive (pages 128–9)

16 Torpedo (pages 108–9)

17 Rowing (pages 144–5)

18 Side plank: star (pages 142–3)

19 Hinge back (thigh stretch) (page 131)

For a **flat stomach,** this is the **workout** for you.

Pilates for bums and thighs

If you want to target tone your body, look no further than this workout. These exercises offer ultimate toning for the thighs and buttocks. Pilates exercises are concentrated on specific muscle groups, so if performed correctly and practised regularly you will reap the rewards in no time.

Start with a few minutes of deep breathing (page 20). Ensure you are standing correctly (page 42) and practise some pliés (page 82). Then continue with your choice of routine. If you have time, spend a few minutes doing some cool down exercises (page 151).

15-minute session

1 Pelvic clocks and tilts (page 27)

2 Starfish (page 54)

3 Spine curls with leg extension (page 101)

4 Hip rolls: feet up (page 61)

5 Leg circles: stage 1 (page 69)

6 The hundred: stage 3 (page 118)

7 Oyster (page 76)

8 Table top (pages 72–3)

9 Cobra (page 104)

30-minute session

1 Pelvic clocks and tilts (page 27)

2 Starfish (page 54)

3 Spine curls with leg extension (page 101)

4 Hip rolls: feet up (page 61)

5 Leg circles: stage 1 (page 69)

6 The hundred: stage 3 (page 118)

7 Coordination (pages 98–9)

8 Oyster (page 76)

9 Side-lying leg kicks: front and back (page 79)

10 Hamstring stretch (page 62)

11 Gluteal stretch (page 81)

12 Table top (pages 72–3)

13 Cobra (page 104)

14 Double leg kick (pages 126–7)

15 Push ups from standing (pages 132–3)

guru guide

• These exercises will tone and strengthen your muscles and give your derrière a lovely shape. Work with precision and you will soon have sculpted, toned buttocks and thighs.

Related exercise for greater impact

Leg circles   Stage 2 (pages 90–1)

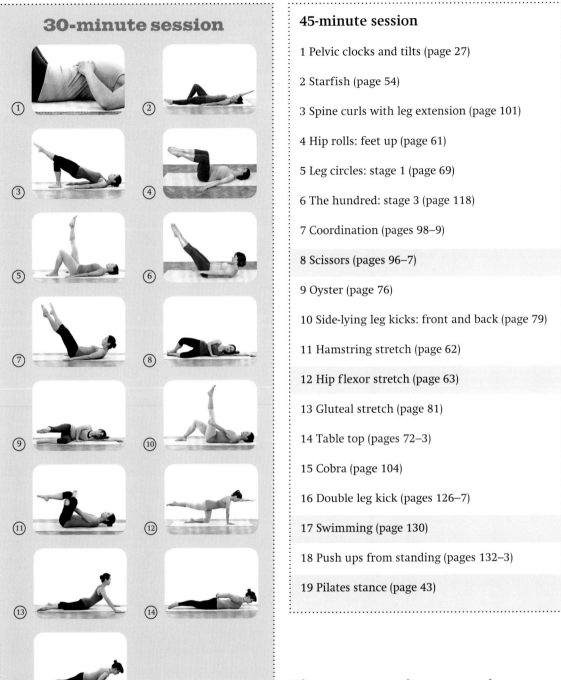

30-minute session

45-minute session

1 Pelvic clocks and tilts (page 27)

2 Starfish (page 54)

3 Spine curls with leg extension (page 101)

4 Hip rolls: feet up (page 61)

5 Leg circles: stage 1 (page 69)

6 The hundred: stage 3 (page 118)

7 Coordination (pages 98–9)

8 Scissors (pages 96–7)

9 Oyster (page 76)

10 Side-lying leg kicks: front and back (page 79)

11 Hamstring stretch (page 62)

12 Hip flexor stretch (page 63)

13 Gluteal stretch (page 81)

14 Table top (pages 72–3)

15 Cobra (page 104)

16 Double leg kick (pages 126–7)

17 Swimming (page 130)

18 Push ups from standing (pages 132–3)

19 Pilates stance (page 43)

These exercises will give your derrière a lovely shape.

Pilates for toned arms

Pilates is fantastic for creating beautifully sculpted limbs, making sure your muscles are strengthened and lengthened, avoiding the stocky muscular look of a body builder. These sessions create a lovely shape to your upper arms so you will be proud to unveil them in vests and T-shirts. This is hard work, so make sure you stretch out afterwards (see page 153).

Start with a few minutes of deep breathing in the relaxation position (pages 20 and 24) and do some pec stretches (page 31). Then continue with your choice of routine. Cool down with floating arms (page 45) and, if you have time, include other cool down exercises (page 151).

15-minute session

1 Arm circles (page 32)

2 Spine curls with arms (page 100)

3 Starfish (page 54)

4 The hundred: stage 1 (page 65)

5 Single leg stretch: stage 1 (page 66)

6 Side plank: star (pages 142–3)

7 Thread the needle (page 110)

8 Swimming (page 130)

9 Push ups from standing (pages 132–3)

30-minute session

1 Arm circles (page 32)

2 Spine curls with arms (page 100)

3 Starfish (page 54)

4 The hundred: stage 1 (page 65)

5 Single leg stretch: stage 1 (page 66)

6 Roll over (pages 124–5)

7 Side plank: star (pages 142–3)

8 Table top (pages 72–3)

9 Cat to down dog (pages 112–13)

10 Thread the needle (page 110)

11 Cobra (page 104)

12 Swimming (page 130)

13 Push ups from standing (pages 132–3)

 guru guide

• To stretch out your triceps (backs of the arms): float one arm above your head. Bend your elbow to release your hand into the centre of your back. Use your other arm to gently press your elbow to deepen the stretch. Repeat on the other side.

Related exercises for greater impact

The hundred	Stages 2/3 (pages 88/118)
Single leg stretch	Stages 2/3 (pages 92–3/117)
Double leg stretch	Stage 2 (pages 120–1)

45-minute session

1 Shoulder drops (page 55)

2 Arm circles (page 32)

3 Spine curls with arms (page 100)

4 Starfish (page 54)

5 The hundred: stage 1 (page 65)

6 Single leg stretch: stage 1 (page 66)

7 Double leg stretch: stage 1 (page 67)

8 Roll over (pages 124–5)

9 Side plank: star (pages 142–3)

10 Table top (page 72–3)

11 Cat to down dog (pages 112–13)

12 Thread the needle (page 110)

13 Cobra (page 104)

14 Swimming (page 130)

15 Swan dive (pages 128–9)

16 Push ups from standing (pages 132–3)

45-minute session

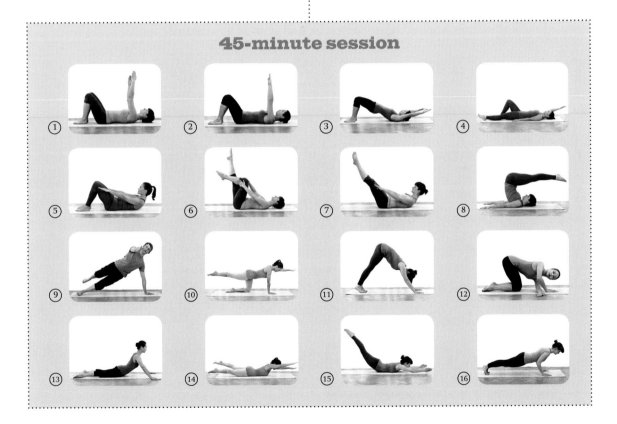

These sessions will beautifully sculpt your arms and shoulders.

Pilates for back strength

Pilates strengthens the deep postural muscles that stabilize your back and pelvis and relaxes muscles that commonly hold on to tension, so all Pilates workouts are strengthening for your spine and will help to alleviate any aches and pains. This session targets the deep stabilizing muscles of the pelvic floor, lower abdominals and the mid-back.

Start with a few minutes of deep breathing (page 20). Ensure you are standing correctly (page 42), then continue with your choice of routine. If you have time, spend a few minutes doing some cool down exercises (page 151).

15-minute session

1 Roll downs (pages 46–7)

2 Side reach (pages 48–9)

3 C-curve (page 39)

4 Spine curls (page 34)

5 The hundred: stage 1 (page 65)

6 Dart with arm circles (pages 106–7)

7 Cobra (page 104)

8 Cat (page 41)

9 Spine stretch forward (page 94)

10 Saw (pages 114–15)

30-minute session

1 Roll downs (pages 46–7)

2 Waist twist: sitting (page 50)

3 C-curve (page 39)

4 Spine curls (page 34)

5 Roll backs (page 71)

6 The hundred: stage 1 (page 65)

7 Rolling like a ball (page 89)

8 Dart with arm circles (pages 106–7)

9 Cobra (page 104)

10 Double leg kick (pages 126–7)

11 Cat (page 41)

12 Spine stretch forward (page 94)

13 Saw (pages 114–15)

14 Kneeling side kicks (pages 134–5)

Pilates strengthens your spine and helps to alleviate any aches and pains.

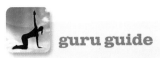
30-minute session

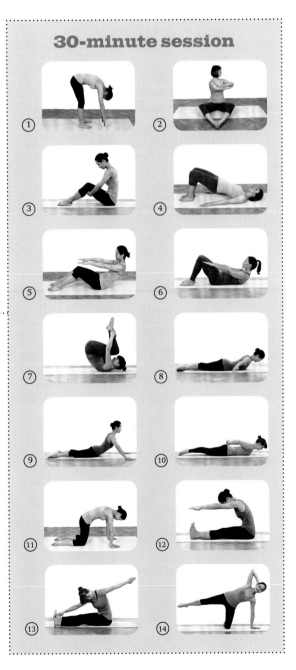

45-minute session

1 Roll downs (pages 46–7)

2 Waist twist: sitting (page 50)

3 C-curve (page 39)

4 Spine curls (page 34)

5 Roll backs (page 71)

6 The hundred: stage 1 (page 65)

7 Rolling like a ball (page 89)

8 Dart with arm circles (pages 106–7)

9 Cobra (page 104)

10 Double leg kick (pages 126–7)

11 Cat (page 41)

12 Spine stretch forward (page 94)

13 Saw (pages 114–15)

14 Kneeling side kicks (pages 134–5)

15 Rowing (pages 144–5)

16 Mermaid (pages 86–7)

17 Hinge back (thigh stretch) (page 131)

18 Table top (pages 72–3)

19 Roll downs (pages 46–7)

20 Standing correctly (page 42)

Related exercises for greater impact

Spine curls	Spine curls: progression (page 100–1)
The hundred	Stages 2/3 (pages 88/118)

Dynamic Pilates for strength

This is a challenging and strengthening workout, showing how Pilates can be effective for building stamina, and making the heart and lungs work hard. You will really get the blood pumping with this one. Link the exercises as swiftly as you can so there is a constant flow of movement and you will enhance its stamina-building potential. This is a particularly challenging combination of exercises, so warm-up effectively (see page 152), and make sure you build up by practising the shorter workouts first.

Start with a few minutes of deep breathing (page 20). Ensure you are standing correctly (page 42), then continue with your choice of routine. If you have time, finish with some cool down exercises (page 151).

15-minute session

1 Roll downs (pages 46–7)

2 Double knee folds (page 35)

3 Spine curls with arms (page 100)

4 Obliques (page 58)

5 The hundred: stage 1 (page 65)

6 Rolling like a ball (page 89)

7 Single leg stretch: stage 1 (page 66)

8 Scissors (pages 96–7)

9 Cobra (page 104)

10 Side-lying leg kicks: front and back (page 79)

11 Push ups from standing (pages 132–3)

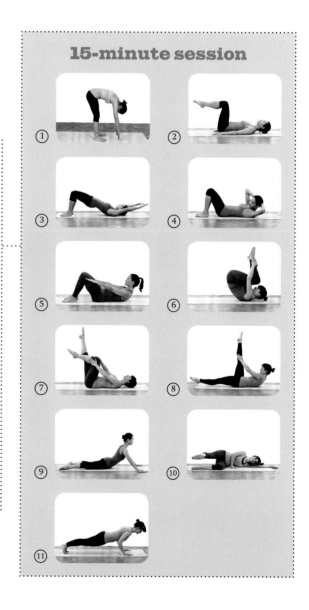

15-minute session

30-minute session

1 Roll downs (pages 46–7)

2 Double knee folds (page 35)

3 Spine curls with arms (page 100)

4 Obliques (page 58)

5 The hundred: stage 1 (page 65)

6 Leg circles: stage 1 (page 69)

7 Rolling like a ball (page 89)

8 Single leg stretch: stage 1 (page 66)

9 Scissors (pages 96–7)

10 Coordination (pages 98–9)

11 Spine stretch forward (page 94)

12 Cobra (page 104)

13 Swimming (page 130)

14 Side-lying leg kicks: front and back (page 79)

15 Push ups from standing (pages 132–3)

Related exercises for greater impact

The hundred	Stages 2/3 (pages 88/118)
Single leg stretch	Stages 2/3 (pages 92–3/117)
Leg circles	Stage 2 (pages 90-1)
Double leg stretch	Stage 2 (pages 120–1)

Link the exercises as swiftly as you can and you will build your stamina.

45-minute session

1 Roll downs (pages 46–7)

2 Double knee folds (page 35)

3 Spine curls with arms (page 100)

4 Obliques (page 58)

5 The hundred: stage 1 (page 65)

6 Leg circles: stage 1 (page 69)

7 Roll up (pages 122–3)

8 Rolling like a ball (page 89)

9 Single leg stretch: stage 1 (page 66)

10 Double leg stretch: stage 1 (page 67)

11 Scissors (pages 96–7)

12 Coordination (pages 98–9)

13 Spine stretch forward (page 94)

14 Saw (pages 114–15)

15 Cobra (page 104)

16 Swan dive (pages 128–9)

17 Swimming (page 130)

18 Side-lying leg kicks: front and back (page 79)

19 The teaser (pages 138–9)

20 Push ups from standing (pages 132–3)

 guru guide

• Before you attempt this session, make sure you have mastered and feel confident with all the exercises, which are mainly intermediate and advanced.

Pilates energy boost

If you are flagging in energy, it's tempting to grab a coffee to give you a temporary rush of energy, or flop onto the sofa and give in to fatigue. Instead, get into the habit of doing some Pilates when you need a boost. This stretches your body, awakens your mind and rejuvenates your limbs, giving you an instant lift, leaving you ready for action.

Start with a few minutes of deep breathing (page 20). Ensure you are standing correctly (page 42), then continue with your choice of routine. Cool down with a few roll downs (pages 46–7) and, if you have time, include other cool down exercises (page 151).

15-minute session

1   Rising on toes (page 44)

2   Roll downs (pages 46–7)

3   Spine curls (page 34)

4   Hip rolls: feet up (page 61)

5   The hundred: stage 1 (page 65)

6   Waist twist (pages 50–1)

7   Dart (page 74)

8   Rest position (page 38)

30-minute session

1   Rising on toes (page 44)

2   Side reach (pages 48–9)

3   Roll downs (pages 46–7)

4   Spine curls (page 34)

5   Hip rolls: feet up (page 61)

6   Curl ups with single knee fold (page 57)

7   The hundred: stage 1 (page 65)

8   Waist twist (pages 50–1)

9   Single leg stretch: stage 1 (page 66)

10 Dart (page 74)

11 Rest position (page 38)

12 Mermaid (pages 86–7)

guru guide

• As you work through these routines remember to always be aware of lengthening through your spine and limbs as you move.

• Pay particular attention to your breath, coordinating your movement in rhythm with your inhalation and exhalation.

Related exercises for greater impact

Rising on toes	Pliés (page 82)
Spine curls	Spine curls: progression (pages 100–1)
The hundred	Stages 2/3 (pages 88–9/118)
Single leg stretch	Stages 2/3 (pages 92–3/119)
Double leg stretch	Stages 2/3 (pages 94–5/120–1)

45-minute session

1 Rising on toes (page 44)

2 Side reach (pages 48–9)

3 Roll downs (pages 46–7)

4 Spine curls (page 34)

5 Hip rolls: feet up (page 61)

6 Curl ups with single knee fold (page 57)

7 Obliques with leg slide (page 59)

8 The hundred: stage 1 (page 65)

9 Waist twist (pages 50–1)

10 Single leg stretch: stage 1 (page 66)

11 Double leg stretch: stage 1 (page 67)

12 Roll backs (pages 70–1)

13 Dart (page 74)

14 Rest position (page 38)

15 Cat (page 41)

16 Mermaid (pages 86–7)

45-minute session

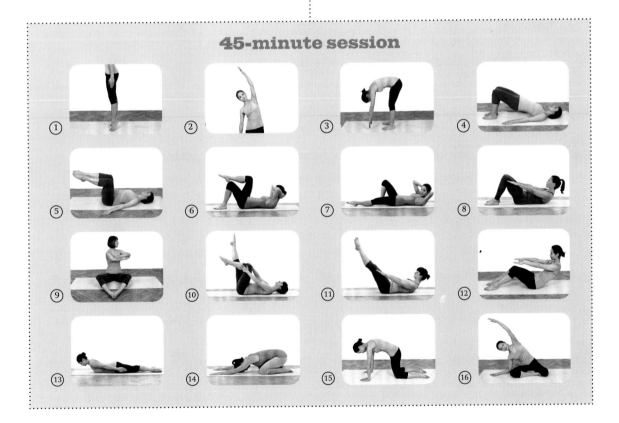

This routine gives you an instant lift, leaving you ready for action.

Pilates desk job reviver

If you have a sedentary job, the chances are your energy levels slump during the day at some point and you experience some stiffness or pain around your neck, lower back or hips. Frequent short breaks for a boost of energy via exercise counter the negative effects of sitting with less-than-perfect posture all day.

It's important to continually think about your posture while you sit at your desk during the day:

Lengthen your neck away from your shoulders, and relax your shoulders into your back.

Check whether your lower spine is curled underneath you and whether you are slumped in your chair. If necessary, place a lumbar support or wedge underneath your sitting bones to encourage you to sit tall and maintain the natural curves of your spine.

Draw your abdominals in and feel supported through the lower back, grow tall through the crown of your head.

Circle your neck, shoulders, ankles and wrists often, to maintain mobility and encourage good circulation.

The exercises opposite are suitable for performing at your office, either standing by your desk, in the toilets or sitting at your desk, without too much embarrassment. You will notice that some of these exercises you have practised so far lying on the mat: here, you can adapt them to perform them sitting at your desk or standing up.

guru guide

• Use these exercises in short bursts throughout the day and you will feel energized and refreshed.

• At the end of each day take some time to release tension and iron out your body by lying in the relaxation position and performing 10–15 minutes of gentle Pilates moves, such as spine curls (page 34), side-lying chest openings (page 80) and hip rolls (pages 60–1).

• Try to get up from your desk once an hour to move around.

Here are a selection of exercises that you can incorporate into your day at intervals, to make sure your body remains supple and stretched and boost your circulation. Take 5 or 10 minutes every couple of hours to perform a few of these exercises and you will feel more alert and less achey throughout the day.

Exercise selection

1 Breathing (page 20)

2 Centring: your pelvic floor (page 26)

3 Arm circles (standing) (page 32)

4 Pliés against a wall (page 83)

5 Rising on toes + floating arms (page 45)

6 Pliés (page 82)

7 Waist twist (sitting or standing) (pages 50–1)

8 Roll downs (pages 46–7)

9 Side reach (sitting or standing) (pages 48–9)

10 Pelvic tilts (page 27)

11 C-curve (page 39)

12 Neck rolls (page 33)

13 Knee folds (sitting at your desk, float knee into chest) (page 35)

14 Hip flexor stretch (standing) (page 63)

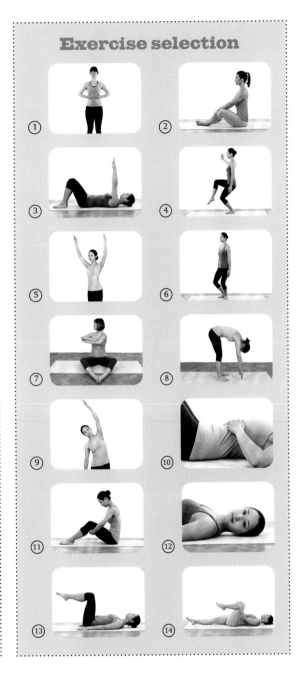

Exercise selection

Continually think about your posture while you sit at your desk.

Pilates for travel and jetlag

When travelling, adjusting to a different time zone is always difficult, and there are often aches and pains from a long flight to contend with. Before you travel, get into the habit of performing this routine at home in the days leading up to your trip. When you arrive at your destination, work through the exercises again to stretch out and release any tension.

Start with a few minutes of deep breathing (page 20). Ensure you are standing correctly (page 42) and do some roll downs (pages 46–7). Then continue with your choice of routine. Cool down in the rest position (page 38) and, if you have time, include other cool down exercises (page 151).

15-minute session

1 Neck rolls (page 33)

2 Shoulder drops (page 55)

3 Spine curls (page 34)

4 Hip rolls: feet down or up (pages 60–1)

5 The hundred: stage 1 (page 65)

6 Cat to down dog (pages 112–13)

7 Cobra (page 104)

8 Thread the needle (page 110)

9 Hamstring stretch (page 62)

10 Hip flexor stretch (page 63)

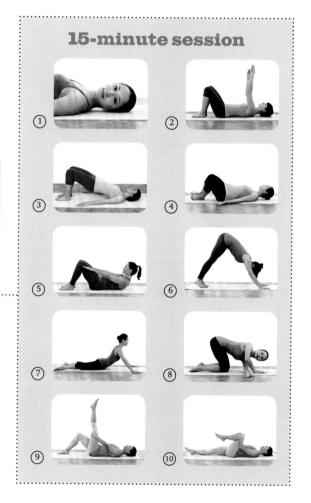

15-minute session

This routine will stretch you out and release any tension.

30-minute session

1 Rising onto toes (page 44)

2 Neck rolls (page 33)

3 Shoulder drops (page 55)

4 Spine curls (page 34)

5 Hip rolls: feet down or up (pages 60–1)

6 The hundred: stage 1 (page 65)

7 Single leg stretch: stage 1 (page 66)

8 Climb a tree (pages 136–7)

9 Cat to down dog (pages 112–13)

10 Cobra (page 104)

11 Table top (pages 72–3)

12 Thread the needle (page 110)

13 Hamstring stretch (page 62)

14 Hip flexor stretch (page 63)

45-minute session

1 Rising onto toes (page 44)

2 Neck rolls (page 33)

3 Shoulder drops (page 55)

4 Spine curls (page 34)

5 Hip rolls: feet down or up (pages 60–1)

6 The hundred: stage 1 (page 65)

7 Single leg stretch: stage 1 (page 66)

8 Climb a tree (pages 136–7)

9 Coordination (pages 98–9)

10 Cat to down dog (pages 112–13)

11 Cobra (page 104)

12 Table top (pages 72–3)

13 Thread the needle (page 110)

14 Spine stretch forward (page 94)

15 The half teaser (pages 102–3)

16 Seal (pages 146–7)

17 Hamstring stretch (page 62)

18 Hip flexor stretch (page 63)

 guru guide

• Try to stay as active as possible on your flight, mobilizing your joints and stretching the body whenever you can.

• It is possible to perform Pilates exercises such as pliés (page 82), roll downs (pages 46–7), side reach (pages 48–9), waist twist (pages 50–1) and neck rolls (page 33) in your seat or in the aisles, to help your circulation and keep you relaxed.

• Stay hydrated by drinking as much water as possible and avoiding alcohol, and you will feel less fatigued on arrival at your destination.

Related exercises for greater impact

Spine curls	Spine curls: progression (pages 100–1)
The hundred	Stages 2/3 (pages 88/118)
Single leg stretch	Stages 2/3 (pages 92–3/117)

Pilates evening wind down

If you need help winding down at the end of a busy day and want to prepare for a restful night's sleep, finishing the day with a Pilates session is a gentle way to ease yourself towards slumber. Make sure the room is quiet or put on some relaxing music, perhaps light some candles or dim the lights. Begin to relax and bring your focus to your body and breath. Lie in the relaxation position (see page 24) and try to let go of any areas of tension, focusing on deeply breathing into your ribcage and softening all stiffness, allowing it to melt away into the mat. Breathe in deeply through your nose, allowing your throat to open. Release the breath in a slow sigh out through your mouth, relaxing the muscles of your face, jaw and neck.

Start with a few minutes of deep breathing in the relaxation position (pages 20 and 24) and do some neck rolls (page 33). Then continue with your choice of routine. Cool down with floating arms (page 45) and, if you have time, include other cool down exercises (page 151).

15-minute session

1 Shoulder drops (page 55)

2 Pelvic clocks (page 27)

3 Spine curls (page 34)

4 Starfish (page 54)

5 Hip rolls: feet down or up (pages 60–1)

6 Knee circles (page 68)

7 Cat (page 41)

8 Cobra (page 104)

9 Side-lying chest openings (page 80)

30-minute session

1 Shoulder drops (page 55)

2 Arm circles (page 32)

3 Pelvic clocks (page 27)

4 Spine curls (page 34)

5 Starfish (page 54)

6 Hip rolls: feet down or up (pages 60–1)

7 Knee circles (page 68)

8 Hamstring stretch (page 62)

9 Cat (page 41)

10 Thread the needle (page 110)

11 Cobra (page 104)

12 Side-lying chest openings (page 80)

13 Mermaid (pages 86–7)

14 Roll downs (pages 46–7)

Finishing the day with a Pilates session is a gentle way to ease yourself towards slumber.

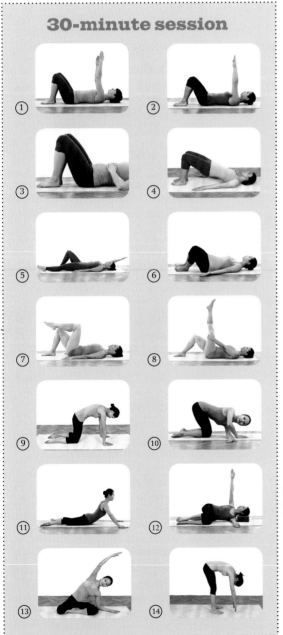

30-minute session

① ② ③ ④ ⑤ ⑥ ⑦ ⑧ ⑨ ⑩ ⑪ ⑫ ⑬ ⑭

45-minute session

1 Shoulder drops (page 55)

2 Arm circles (page 32)

3 Pelvic clocks (page 27)

4 Knee drops (page 29)

5 Spine curls (page 34)

6 Starfish (page 54)

7 Hip rolls: feet down or up (pages 60–1)

8 Knee circles (page 68)

9 Hamstring stretch (page 62)

10 Hip flexor stretch (page 63)

11 Gluteal stretch (page 81)

12 Cat (page 41)

13 Thread the needle (page 110)

14 Cobra (page 104)

15 Side-lying chest openings (page 80)

16 Mermaid (pages 86–7)

17 Roll downs (pages 46–7)

guru guide

• Focus on your breath, allowing your breathing to become steadily deeper and your exhalation long and slow. This will help you to relax and prepare for sleep.

• Perform the moves slowly and precisely, and allow your body to relase all tension.

Index

A

alignment 19
arm circles 32

B

breathing 16
  controlling 20

C

c-curve 39
cat 41
cat to down dog 112–13
centring 16, 26
challenging muscles exercises
  c-curve 39
  cat 41
  cat to down dog 112–13
  centring 26
  climb a tree 136–7
  cobra 37, 104
  coordination 98–9
  criss cross 140–1
  curl ups 56–7
  dart 74
  dart with arm circles 106–7
  double leg kick 126–7
  double leg lifts 105
  double leg stretch 67, 120–1
  half teaser 102–3
  hinge back (thigh stretch) 131
  hundred 65, 88, 118
  knee folds 35
  kneeling side kicks 134–5
  leg circles 69, 90–1
  obliques 58–9
  oyster 76–7
  prone leg lifts 75
  push ups from standing 132–3
  roll backs 70–1
  roll over 124–5
  roll up 122–3
  rolling like a ball 89
  rowing 144–5
  saw 114–15
  scissors 96–7
  seal 146–7

side plank: star 142–3
side-lying leg kicks 78–9
single leg stretch 66, 92–3, 119
spine curls 100–1
spine stretch forward 94
spine twist 95
swan dive 128–9
swimming 130
table top 72–3
teaser 138–9
thread the needle 110–111
torpedo 108–9
chin tucks 33
climb a tree 136–7
cobra 104
  preparation 37
concentration 17
control 17
cooling down 151
cooling down exercises
  arm circles 32
  centring 26
  chin tucks 33
  floating arms 45
  gluteal stretch 81
  hamstring stretch 62
  hip flexor stretch 63
  neck rolls 33
  neutral pelvis and spine 24
  pec stretch 31
  pelvic clocks 27
  pelvic tilts 27
  Pilates stance 43
  pliés 82–3
  relaxation position 24
  rest position 38
  rising on toes 44
  roll downs 46, 47
  shoulder drops 55
  side-lying chest openings 80
  spine curls 34
  standing correctly 42
  starfish 54
  waist twist 50–1
coordination 98–9
criss cross 140–1
curl ups 56–7
  with single knee fold 57

D

dart 74
  with arm circles 106–7
double leg kick 126–7
double leg lifts 105
double leg stretch
  stage 1 67
  stage 2 120–1

F

floating arms 45
four-point kneeling 40

G

gluteal stretch 81

H

half teaser 102–3
hamstring stretch 62
hinge back (thigh stretch) 131
hip flexor stretch 63
hip rolls
  feet down 60
  feet up 61
hundred
  preparation 64
  stage 1 65
  stage 2 88
  stage 3 118

J

joint mobility exercises
  arm circles 32
  cat to down dog 112–13
  climb a tree 136–7
  coordination 98–9
  criss cross 140–1
  dart with arm circles 106–7
  double leg kick 126–7
  double leg lifts 105
  floating arms 45
  half teaser 102–3
  hinge back (thigh stretch)
    131

hundred 118
knee circles 68
knee drops 29
knee folds 35
kneeling side kicks 134–5
leg circles 69, 90–1
leg slides 28
oyster 76–7
pliés 82–3
prone leg lifts 75
push ups from standing
    132–3
ribcage closure 30
rising on toes 44
roll over 124–5
roll up 122–3
rowing 144–5
scissors 96–7
seal 146–7
shoulder drops 55
side plank: star 142–3
side-lying leg kicks 78–9
single leg stretch 92–3, 119
spine curls 100–1
starfish 54
swimming 130
table top 72–3
teaser 138–9
torpedo 108–9
joints, warming up 151

K

knee circles 68
knee drops 29
knee folds 35
kneeling side kicks 134–5

L

leg circles
    stage 1 69
    stage 2 90–1
leg slides 28

M

mermaid 86–7
movement 16
muscles, challenging 152; see
    also challenging muscles
    exercises

N

neck rolls 33
neutral pelvis and spine 25

O

obliques 58–9
    with leg slide 59
oyster 76–7
    with foot lift 77
    with leg extension 77

P

pec stretch 31
pelvic clocks 27
pelvic floor, centring, see centring
pelvic tilts 27
Pilates sessions, see sessions
Pilates stance 43
Pilates
    benefits of 17
    introducing 7
    origins 15
    principles 16–17
Pilates, Joe
    and alignment 19
    and breathing 16, 20
    and centring 16, 26
    classical repertoire 128, 138, 144
    and spine 18
    teachings 15
pliés 82
    against a wall 83
posture 21
precision 16
prone leg lifts 75
prone stabilizing 36
push ups from standing 132–3

R

relaxation position 24
rest position 38
ribcage closure 30
rising on toes 44
rising on toes + floating arms 45
roll backs 70–1
roll downs
    against the wall 46
    freestanding 47
roll over 124–5

roll up 122–3
rolling like a ball 89
rowing 144–5

S

saw 114–15
scissors 96–7
seal 146–7
sessions
    for abdominals 156–7
    for back strength 162–3
    for bums and thighs 158–9
    desk job reviver 168–9
    energy boost 166–7
    evening wind down 172–3
    for posture 154–5
    for strength 164–5
    for toned arms 160–1
    for travel and jetlag 170–1
shoulder drops 55
side plank: star 142–3
side reach
    kneeling 48
    standing 49
side-lying chest openings 80
side-lying leg kicks 78–9
    front and back 79
    lift and lower 78–9
single leg stretch
    stage 1 66
    stage 2 92–3
    stage 3 119
spinal mobility
    c-curve 39
    cat 41
    cat to down dog 112–13
    cobra 37, 104
    coordination 98–9
    criss cross 140–1
    curl ups 56–7
    dart 74
    dart with arm circles 106–7
    double leg kick 126–7
    half teaser 102–3
    hip rolls 60–1
    hundred 65, 88, 118
    mermaid 86–7
    obliques 58–9
    roll backs 70–1
    roll downs 46, 47
    roll over 124–5

spinal mobility (cont.)
  roll up 122–3
  rolling like a ball 89
  saw 114–15
  scissors 96–7
  seal 146–7
  side reach 48–9
  side-lying chest openings 80
  single leg stretch 119
  spine curls 34, 100–1
  spine stretch forward 94
  spine twist 95
  swan dive 128–9
  swimming 130
  teaser 138–9
  thread the needle 110–111
  waist twist 50–1
spine curls 34
  with arms 100
  with leg extension 101
  progressions 100–1
spine stretch forward 94
spine
  mobilizing 150
  movements of 18
spine twist 95
standing correctly 42
starfish 54
stretches
  dynamic 153
  static 153
stretching exercises
  cat to down dog 112–13
  climb a tree 136–7
  criss cross 140–1
  double leg kick 126–7

double leg stretch 67, 120–1
gluteal stretch 81
hamstring stretch 62
hinge back (thigh stretch) 131
hip flexor stretch 63
pec stretch 31
push ups from standing 132–3
roll over 124–4
rowing 144–5
saw 114–15
scissors 96–7
side reach 48–9
single leg stretch 66, 92–3, 119
spine stretch forward 94
thread the needle 110–111
stretching out 153
swan dive 128–9
swimming 130
symmetry 19

T
table top 72–3
teaser 138–9
thread the needle 110–11
  with arm openings 111
torpedo 108–9

W
waist twist
  sitting 50
  standing 51
warming up 150
warming-up exercises
  arm circles 32

c-curve 39
cat 41
centring 26
chin tucks 33
floating arms 45
four-point kneeling 40
gluteal stretch 81
hamstring stretch 62
hip flexor stretch 63
hip rolls 60–1
hundred preparation 64
knee circles 68
knee drops 29
knee folds 35
leg slides 28
neck rolls 33
neutral pelvis and spine 25
pec stretch 31
pelvic clocks 27
pelvic tilts 27
Pilates stance 43
pliés 82–3
prone stabilizing 36
relaxation position 24
rest position 38
ribcage closure 30
rising on toes 44
roll downs 46, 47
shoulder drops 55
side reach 48–9
side-lying chest openings 80
spine curls 34
standing correctly 42
starfish 54
waist twist 50–1
workouts, structuring 150–3

Acknowledgments

There are many people who deserve huge thanks for ensuring *My Pilates Guru* came into existence. Firstly and most importantly, to the wonderful teaching team at Body Control Pilates in London where I trained, who are a continual source of inspiration for the never-ending learning on my own Pilates journey, and to my fantastic teachers over the years, Victoria Hodgson at Body Control and Deborah Henley at The Pilates Room, for encouraging me to push my own body and understanding to its limits and beyond in order to strengthen and progress. Thanks also go to my lovely husband who has been a Pilates guinea pig on many an occasion without ever complaining. Thanks to the Octopus editorial and production team and, in particular, to Emma Callery for her patience and diligence in bringing the book to its completion.

Credits

My Pilates Guru created for Octopus Publishing Group Ltd by:

Managing editor: Emma Callery
Designer: Alison Shackleton
Photographer: Nikki English

Models: Lucy Anderson, Simon Lindsay, Jacqueline Pegg, Katherine Pentecost, Sharon Wu
Hair and make-up: Anne-Marie Simak